BASIC SURGICAL OPERATIONS

Commissioning Editor: Laurence Hunter
Project Development Manager: Janice Urquhart
Project Manager: Frances Affleck
Design direction: Erik Bigland
Illustrated by: Adrian Shaw, Jan Sharp

BASIC SURGICAL OPERATIONS

M. E. Foster MChir FRCS

Consultant Surgeon,
Royal Glamorgan Hospital,
Ynysmaerdy, Llantrisant, Wales;
External Professor, University of Glamorgan, Wales

G. Morris-Stiff FRCS

Research Fellow,
Welsh Transplantation Research Group,
Department of Surgery,
University of Wales College of Medicine,
Cardiff, Wales

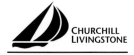

CHURCHILL
LIVINGSTONE

EDINBURGH LONDON NEW YORK PHILADELPHIA ST LOUIS SYDNEY TORONTO 2000

CHURCHILL LIVINGSTONE
An imprint of Harcourt Publishers Limited

© Harcourt Publishers Limited 2000

First published 2000

ISBN 0443 063591

British Library of Cataloguing in Publication Data
A catalogue record for this book is available from the
British Library.

Library of Congress Cataloging in Publication Data
A catalog record for this book is available from the Library
of Congress.

Medical knowledge is constantly changing. As
information becomes available, changes in treatment,
procedures, equipment and the use of drugs become
necessary. The author and publisher have, as far as it is
possible, taken care to ensure that the information given
in the text is accurate and up-to-date. However, readers
are strongly advised to confirm that the information,
especially with regard to drug usage, complies with
current legislation and standards of practice.

The
publisher's
policy is to use
**paper manufactured
from sustainable forests**

Typeset by IMH(Cartrif), Loanhead, Scotland
Printed in China

A training in surgery is very much an apprenticeship and requires the trainee to spend long periods in the operating theatre, observing what is done and assisting other surgeons to do it. When it is judged your time to perform the operation you will be assisted by someone more senior for the first few occasions. After that you may well be on your own and although you will be familiar with the basic manoeuvres of the operation, there will be nobody to remind you of the order in which they are done and to point out the tricks which can make the operation easier to perform. Our book is an attempt to remedy this by serving as an aide memoire to which you can refer before commencing an operation.

Very few of the procedures are original for they have been accrued over many years from colleagues, both senior and junior. Nor are these operations exclusive, for there are many variations that give just as good results. The techniques described here are those that we have come to prefer and continue to practise.

Unlike other books on operative surgery, this one is designed to be portable to allow you to carry it on your person whilst going about your daily duties. To achieve this goal, the text has been kept to a minimum and only the more important aspects of each operation are discussed. As a consequence the diagnostic features of the condition and appropriate preoperative investigations, although important, have been omitted.

The scope of the book is aimed to cover the period from the first basic surgical training post up to the third year of the specialist registrar training. As such it covers many operations regarded by the trainee as being mundane but which are often poorly performed.

We have chosen not to include proprietary names of sutures or eponymous instruments (unless one is invaluable) as there are many alternatives available.

M. E. Foster
G. Morris-Stiff   2000

ACKNOWLEDGEMENTS

We are indebted to Miss Nicola Richardson for typing the manuscript and to Professor Leslie Hughes and his care and attention to detail in proofreading the text.

We also wish to thank Professor John Salaman, joint author of the forerunner of this book, who has encouraged us to produce this updated version.

Finally we would like to acknowledge the hard work of Janice Sharp and Adrian Shaw, the two medical artists who have been responsible for all the illustrations.

CONTENTS

CONTENTS

1

INS AND OUTS

Convention would have it that body hair is removed from the operative field prior to surgery both for aesthetic reasons and to allow a clear surface for the application of adhesive dressings. The shaving should ideally be performed on the morning of surgery by trained nursing staff and care must be taken not to cause cuts or abrasions as these predispose to infection.

peasing in appearance etc.

The two commonest agents for skin preparation are chlorhexidine (0.5%) and alcoholic betadine (1% povidine iodine in 70% alcohol). These are applied to the operative fields and a wide margin surrounding this area in case there is a need to extend or vary the incision peroperatively.

Having prepared the area for surgery the region must be appropriately draped. This may be done either with sterile linen drapes or with disposable fabrics. The latter have the advantage of being impermeable and waterproof, thus reducing the risk of contamination by the surgeon; however, they are significantly more expensive. Polyurethane incisable drapes enjoy widespread usage in orthopaedic and vascular surgery and amongst some general surgeons. Their use is again limited by cost.

The requirement of any incision is that it provides good access with a low failure rate whilst at the same time being cosmetically acceptable. The correct choice of incision is one that gives the best exposure for a particular operation. There are therefore many ways of entering the peritoneal cavity depending upon the organ being treated and the particular operation being performed.

The main abdominal incisions for elective surgery are shown below.

hernia through a Kocher's incision is very difficult to cure.

In the case of emergency laparotomy where the diagnosis is not obvious, a midline incision is preferable, centred on the umbilicus (the 'incision of indecision' or registrar's incision). This can then simply be extended up or down, depending on the findings, to give optimal access.

Having chosen the appropriate incision, divide the skin and subcutaneous tissues, avoiding multiple

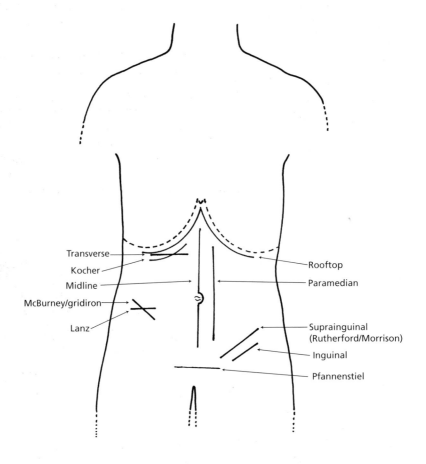

Transverse
Kocher
Midline
McBurney/gridiron
Lanz
Rooftop
Paramedian
Suprainguinal (Rutherford/Morrison)
Inguinal
Pfannenstiel

Fig. 1.1

Midline incisions allow rapid access, with minimal blood loss and easy closure. Paramedian incisions take longer to form and close and may be associated with a slightly higher blood loss but they have a low complication rate. Transverse incisions may be muscle-cutting (e.g. Kocher) or muscle-splitting (e.g. Lanz) but despite providing good access they take longer to perform, have an increased blood loss and a higher complication rate – an incisional

slices into the fat as this may lead to necrosis. It is often helpful to lift the skin edges as you cut down to the aponeurosis.

In the case of a midline incision, the midline can be recognised by the presence of interdigitating fibres that become visible as the fat is cleared away. Divide the linea alba for the full length of the skin incision.

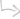

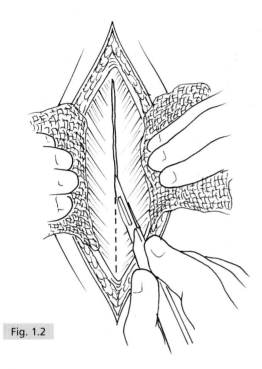

Fig. 1.2

Pick up the peritoneum between clips and confirm by palpation that no bowel is adherent, then nick the peritoneum between the clips.

Insert a finger beneath the wound to ensure no underlying adhesions, then divide the peritoneum carefully with scissors, again for the full length of the incision.

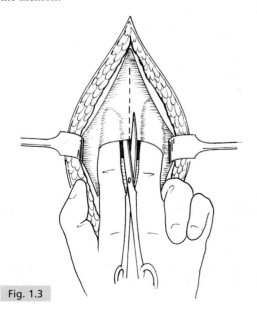

Fig. 1.3

It is important to ensure that there are no adherent viscera. In the lower midline care must be taken to avoid the bladder.

It is crucial that haemostasis is achieved at every stage of the incision.

For paramedian incisions, incise the skin approximately 4 cm from the midline and, after incising the anterior rectus sheath, ask the assistant to hold up the medial edge vertically with three or four clips. With the aid of a scalpel, divide the sheath from the muscle at the points of its intersections. Reflect the rectus laterally to allow access to the posterior rectus sheath. Incise the posterior sheath for the full length of the wound and then divide the peritoneum.

For a subcostal incision, keep parallel and approximately 2 cm from the costal margin. Divide the anterior rectus sheath and pass a long forceps under the muscle to emerge at the midline. This allows you to pull a swab back under the muscle to protect underlying structures from the cutting diathermy as the muscle is divided.

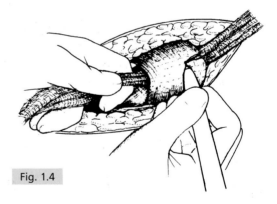

Fig. 1.4

A small incision is then made in the peritoneum, allowing access of one or two fingers. This allows protection of underlying viscera whilst the transversus abdominis muscle is divided.

Better to cut in direction of muscle or 90° to muscle?

An exploratory laparotomy should be performed before every abdominal procedure. It is worth being diligent, as unexpected pathology can often turn up. Start at the oesophageal hiatus and follow an anticlockwise spiral.

Feel the distal oesophagus and stomach. Look at and feel the duodenum. Palpate the liver, gallbladder and right kidney. Move down along the right colon to the caecum and then put a hand in the pelvis. Move up the sigmoid colon to the descending colon and, upon reaching the splenic flexure, palpate the spleen and left kidney. Complete the outer circuit by palpating along the transverse colon and don't forget the pancreas and aorta. Next move on to the small bowel and the inner circuit. Commence at the ligament of Treitz and carefully palpate along the length of the jejunum and ileum until you reach the caecum.

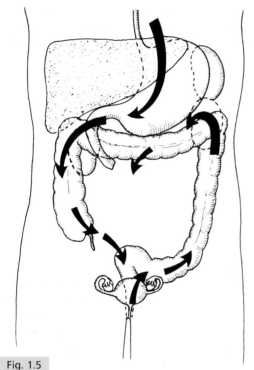

Fig. 1.5

The laparotomy circuit

Midline

A 'mass-suture' technique incorporating both peritoneum and linea alba is commonly performed and is quicker and just as effective as closure of individual layers so long as certain rules are obeyed. The suture should be either a size 0 or 1 non-absorbable suture and may be either a loop or single-stranded. Take bites at 1 cm intervals, each bite taken 1 cm from the wound edge, and passing vertically through the abdominal wall. Using this technique the length of suture utilised should be at least four times the length of the wound (Jenkins' rule).

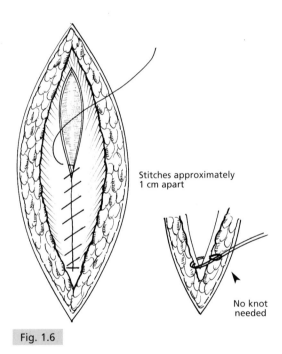

Stitches approximately 1 cm apart

No knot needed

Fig. 1.6

Having completed the suturing it is desirable to bury the knot to prevent irritation.

Paramedian

Close the peritoneum, using an absorbable size 1 suture. A simple over-and-over technique is all that is required. The anterior rectus sheath is then closed as for a midline incision, again applying Jenkins' rule.

Tension sutures

Classical all-layer sutures incorporating rubber or plastic sleeves are inefficient, can damage the skin and are cosmetically unacceptable; they are therefore best avoided. Patients who are debilitated, malnourished, distended or taking steroids can have their wound strengthened with interrupted double near-and-far sutures as described by Professor L.E. Hughes.

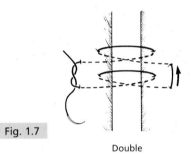

Fig. 1.7

Double

These should be fashioned from size 1/0 or 2/0 non-absorbable sutures and placed in the anterior rectus sheath or linea alba every few centimetres for the entire length of the wound. All double near-and-far sutures should be in place prior to closure with a standard continuous non-absorbable suture. As the continuous suture ascends the wound, the near-and-far sutures are tied to reinforce the wound.

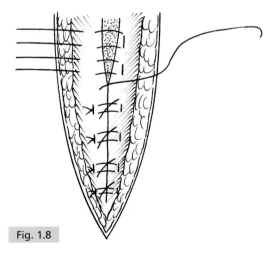

Fig. 1.8

Closing with continuous loop nylon and double near-and-far sutures

INS AND OUTS

Skin closure

There are many different ways of closing skin incisions and each surgeon has their own favourite technique. For the majority of wounds, a subcuticular closure may be adopted and offers good cosmetic results. An undyed absorbable size 2/0 suture is preferable as this does not have to be removed and does not tattoo the skin.

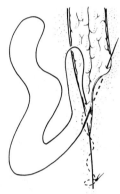

Fig. 1.9

Subcuticular closure

Alternatives include a subcuticular non-absorbable beaded suture or skin staples.

For small wounds interrupted sutures may be utilised. These include simple interrupted, vertical mattress and horizontal mattress sutures.

Key points

1. Make sure the patient is lying symmetrically on the operating table before starting the incision.
2. If previous incisions are present try to enter the abdominal cavity through a new site.
3. Make full use of the length of the incision and do not be afraid to increase the length of the incision should this become necessary. Big complications can occur through small holes!
4. Good exposure is the secret to success, so do not proceed with the operation until you have secured haemostasis and have sufficient retractors to display the operative field.
5. Before closing the skin it is worth infiltrating under both the rectus sheath and skin with 0.25% bupivicaine to reduce postoperative pain.
6. If wound closure is a struggle, check with the anaesthetist that the patient is fully relaxed.

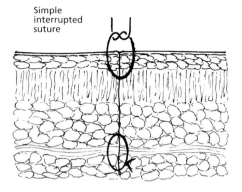

Simple interrupted suture

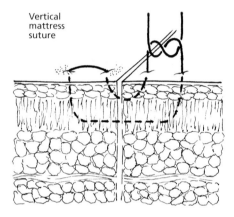

Vertical mattress suture

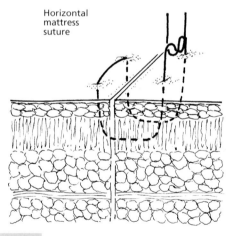

Horizontal mattress suture

Fig. 1.10

The essential components of laparoscopy are:

1. Establishment and maintenance of a pneumoperitoneum.
2. Insertion of trocars.
3. Inspection of the peritoneal cavity.
4. Removal of trocars and closure of wounds.

Establishment and maintenance of a pneumoperitoneum

A pneumoperitoneum can be established by one of two methods:

Closed laparoscopy with Veress needle

Before commencing surgery place the patient in the Trendelenburg position to tip the bowel away from the pelvis. Using a scalpel make a 1–2 cm infraumbilical incision (either transverse or vertical) and deepen it down to the rectus sheath.

Whilst holding up the abdominal wall, carefully insert a Veress needle perpendicularly until you feel it 'give' as it enters the peritoneal cavity. When the 'give' is felt alter the needle's trajectory so that it is pointing at about 45° towards the pelvis.

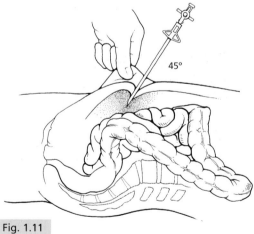

Fig. 1.11

Use either the saline drip test to demonstrate satisfactory insertion, or aspiration test to confirm no return.

Open laparoscopy with Hassan cannula

Through a similar incision pick up and incise the rectus sheath. Place stay sutures on each side of the linea alba.

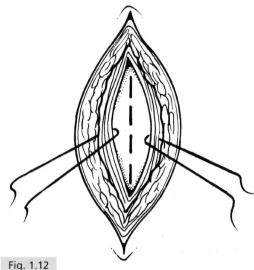

Fig. 1.12

Incise the peritoneum and enter the peritoneal cavity under direct vision. Insert a finger and sweep away any adhesions directly under the incision. Insert the port and use the stay sutures to hold the port in place.

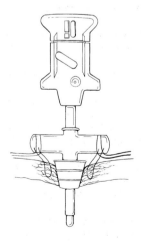

Fig. 1.13

This technique can be used routinely but is particularly useful in the presence of previous abdominal surgery. Slowly insufflate with CO_2 (1 L/min), watching that the intra-abdominal pressure does not exceed 0–5 mmHg. Percuss the abdomen to ensure symmetrical abdominal distension. Increase the flow if all the above are satisfactory, maintaining a pressure of about 13–15 mmHg. The total volume of gas varies but 4–5 L usually suffices.

Check for correct positioning by releasing the gas tap or valve and hearing CO_2 leak from the peritoneal cavity. Attach the laparoscope and camera. If the trocar site is seen to be bleeding local pressure may be sufficient. Alternatively, introduce a suture on a large hand needle and ligate the vessel at the bleeding point.

If bleeding persists insert a Foley catheter, inflate the balloon and hold under traction.

Trocar insertion

Insertion of the first port in a closed pneumoperitoneum is a potentially dangerous procedure that is eliminated when the open method is chosen.

A 10 mm disposable cannula is preferred for initial placement in the umbilicus. Introduce the cannula using a corkscrew technique aiming slightly towards the pelvis. Place your index finger along the length of the trocar so as to prevent accidental over-insertion and damage to underlying viscera.

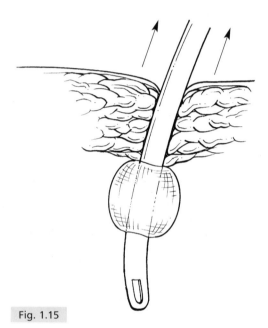

Fig. 1.15

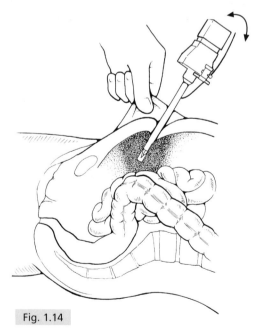

Fig. 1.14

Inspection of peritoneal cavity

Having established a pneumoperitoneum, perform a thorough inspection of the peritoneal cavity. Insert a second port under direct vision in an appropriate position depending upon the area under inspection. A 5 mm cannula placed in the epigastric region will usually suffice. Through this cannula insert a forceps to allow you to gently manipulate the viscera so as to allow a complete laparoscopy. If a biopsy is required the forceps may be removed and a pair of scissors with diathermy inserted to obtain a tissue sample.

Removal of trocars and closure of wounds

Remove the trocars under direct vision, taking care to check for port-site haemostasis. The umbilical and epigastric port-sites should be closed formally using an absorbable suture, e.g. J-shaped absorbable suture. Skin closure is by tapes or sutures. Always infiltrate the wound using bupivacaine as this assists postoperative analgesia.

Key points

1. Always check the instruments thoroughly before commencing laparoscopy.
2. Always check that a pneumoperitoneum has been established before inserting a trocar.
3. Watch out for leaks via taps or umbilical incision, in particular if the Hassan technique is used. You may need to purse-string the umbilicus to get a good seal.
4. An accidental insufflation of the rectus sheath is recognised by an increase in inflation pressure and an asymmetrical distension of the abdomen. If this occurs simply stop insufflation, reposition the Veress needle and restart the insufflation.
5. Always warm the telescope before inserting it in order to prevent misting.
6. Never place the light cable on the drapes as it is very hot and may burn the patient.
7. If you are assisting in a laparoscopic procedure as the camera operator, make sure all your movements are smooth or they may induce 'sea sickness'.
8. If blood obscures the lens try wiping the lens on the omentum. If this fails to clear the view, remove the telescope and clean the lens with an anti-fog wipe.

DIATHERMY

Diathermy is a very quick and useful way of obtaining haemostasis. Diathermy relies on the principle that when current passes through a conductor some of the electrical energy is turned to thermal energy (heat). The amount of heat generated is inversely proportional to the volume of tissue traversed by the current – hence the importance of broad contact with the diathermy pad.

There are two types of commercially available diathermy: namely, monopolar and bipolar.

Monopolar diathermy

Monopolar diathermy is the form most familiar to surgeons and consists of an electrode capable of producing a high current density, a patient plate and a dispersive cable.

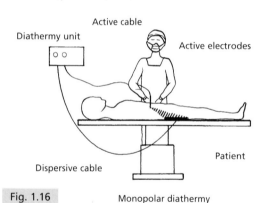

Fig. 1.16   Monopolar diathermy

Monopolar diathermy may be used to either cut or coagulate tissue. Cutting is most effective when the electrode is placed a small distance away from the tissues. In this scenario a continuous current leads to electrical discharge across an air gap, creating high-temperature sparks which cause cellular water to explode. If a monopolar diathermy in cutting mode is touched against tissue the current is less intense and instead causes dehydration and protein denaturation. When coagulation is selected, tissue damage occurs by a process known as 'fulguration' (fulgurate = to flash like lightening). A coagulating current consists of a sine-wave energy supplied in

bursts with high peak voltages. Since the current is turned off for a significant period of the time when the diathermy is set to coagulation less electrical energy is applied to the tissues. A combination of the two effects leads to a blended current.

Bipolar diathermy

With this form of diathermy the current transfer occurs between the tips of two small electrodes and is therefore not dispersed through the patient.

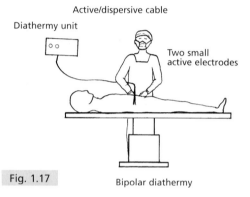

Fig. 1.17   Bipolar diathermy

Bipolar diathermy is safer, as the current only flows between the tips of the active electrodes and is therefore preferred in some paediatric surgical operations. However, it is only able to coagulate and is unable to cut tissue effectively.

Key points

1. Always supervise and ensure correct placement of the pad. This is the legal responsibility of the surgeon and not the scrub nurse.
2. Ensure that the machine is serviced as for manufacturer's recommendations. Despite built-in safety devices burns can still occur.
3. If the patient has a pacemaker, try and avoid monopolar diathermy. If it must be used place the plate as far as possible from the pacemaker and carefully monitor the heart rate.
4. There is potential for alcohol-based cleaning preparations to ignite and set fire to drapes – therefore excess solutions should not be allowed to pool on the drapes.
5. Do not try and diathermy a bleeding point on something that has a long pedicle, e.g. testis, as current will cause it to heat up and may cause thrombosis of the vessels.
6. Never activate the diathermy until the tip of the instrument has reached the desired position. In open surgery the diathermy is kept in an insulated quiver; however, in laparoscopic surgery the tip may still be in the operating field and cause inadvertent burning.
7. In laparoscopic diathermy always check the insulation for cracks, as these may expose the active electrode and lead to accidental burning out of sight of the operative field.
8. Direct coupling (instrument to instrument) occurs in laparoscopic surgery if your diathermy is in contact with a second instrument when the pedal is activated and may lead to unrecognised tissue damage. Capacitance coupling is a phenomenon occurring around the trocar site when trocar materials are alternated between plastic sleeve and a metal port. The insertion of a diathermy creates a capacitor which stores electrical charge before discharging it to the surrounding skin.
9. A further risk in laparoscopic surgery is with retained heat. To avoid burns never let the tip rest on tissue and try to remove the instrument when it is not in use.

2

LUMPS, BUMPS AND OTHERS

EXCISION OF SKIN LESIONS

Indications

1. Any lesion believed to be malignant.
2. In cases of diagnostic dilemma.
3. Cosmesis.

Setting up

1. Local anaesthetic: 0.5–1% lignocaine with or without 1 in 100,000 adrenaline depending upon the site of the lesion. Adrenaline should be avoided in the case of surgery on the fingers, ears and penis.

Procedure

Introduce the local anaesthetic both intradermally and subcutaneously around the lesion, keeping the needle very superficial to start with and then working deeper. Use a small scalpel blade (size 10 or 15) and, holding the knife near to the vertical, make an elliptical incision around the lesion and then incise under the lesion to remove it.

It is important to incise in the direction of Langer's lines, in particular for head and lesions so as to ensure good cosmesis.

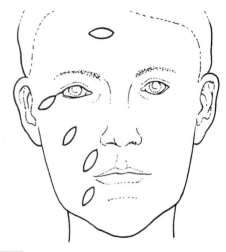

Fig. 2.2

Close the skin with an undyed subcutaneous non-absorbable suture.

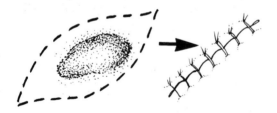

Fig. 2.1

Key points

1. For suspected basal and squamous carcinomas ensure that the whole lesion is excised.
2. Always orientate the specimen by placing a suture in one end and drawing an annotated diagram for the pathologist as this will aid comment on the completeness of excision.
3. For suspected melanomas the margin of normal skin removed should be proportional to the estimated thickness of the lesion: a 1 cm margin for a 1 mm lesion, a 2 cm margin for a 2 mm lesion and a 3 cm margin for a 3 mm lesion. Hence it is important to obtain histological confirmation by incisional biopsy prior to excising a lesion believed to be a melanoma. In addition, larger melanomas should be excised under general anaesthetic.

Indications

Cosmetic.

Setting up

1. Local or general anaesthetic depending upon the site and size of the lipoma.
2. Position dependent upon position of the lesion.

Procedure

Make an incision over the lesion along Langer's lines.

Deepen the incision using the blades of a pair of scissors to develop a plane between the capsule and surrounding adipose tissue.

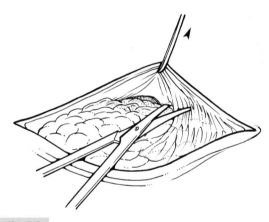

Fig. 2.3

Use a finger to 'winkle' out the lipoma.

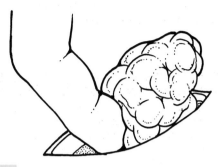

Fig. 2.4

Control any bleeding points with diathermy or fine absorbable sutures.

Obliterate the dead space with a couple of interrupted absorbable sutures and close the skin with interrupted absorbable sutures.

Key points

1. In order to minimise the length of the incision, make a 2–3 cm cut in the skin and incise into the capsule. Then use the 'squeeze' technique to expel the lipoma by applying pressure to the lipoma between finger and thumb.
2. If bleeding occurs do not be afraid to insert a small suction drain.

Indications

1. Cosmetic.
2. Complications – recurrent infections, sebaceous horn.

Setting up

1. Local anaesthetic: 1% lignocaine with or without 1 in 100,000 adrenaline (see Excision of Skin Lesions, p. 16).

Procedure

Introduce the local anaesthetic around the lesion. Make an elliptical incision over the top of the cyst to include the punctum if visible.

Fig. 2.5

Grasp the cyst by the skin ellipse and carefully dissect on either side to free the cyst from surrounding fat and subcutaneous tissue.

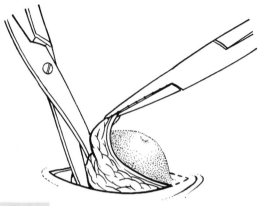

Fig. 2.6

Close the skin with size 2/0 or 3/0 interrupted non-absorbable sutures.

Key points

1. If the cyst ruptures, carefully swab away the debris and ensure that all the remaining cyst wall is removed. Failure to do this may result in cyst recurrence.
2. If the cyst is clearly infected, it may either be drained, excised and the wound left open, or the operation may be postponed until the infection has settled. Infected cysts are harder to excise and tend to be bloodier than non-infected cysts.

Indications

To confirm the cause of lymphadenopathy when clinical examination and investigations (including FNA – fine needle aspiration) have failed to establish the diagnosis.

Setting up

1. General or local anaesthetic.
2. Supine position.

Procedure

The site of incision will depend on the precise location of the lymphadenopathy. The biopsy incision should be such that it will be encompassed by the incision of a radical procedure should this prove necessary.

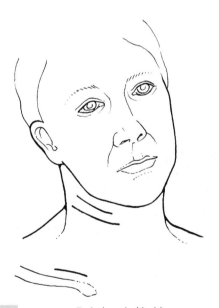

Fig. 2.7   Typical cervical incision

Deepen the incision by opening the blades of a pair of dissecting scissors. Identify the lymph node and carefully apply a pair of tissue forceps. Complete the dissection and identify the pedicle, which usually contains a small artery.

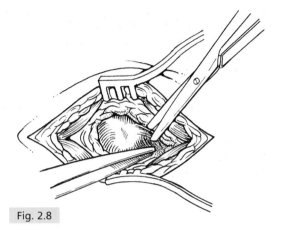

Fig. 2.8

Use either diathermy or a fine tie to control the vessel. Excise the lymph node and send it for histological examination.

Ensure haemostasis and close the wound with interrupted absorbable sutures and a subcuticular suture for the skin.

Key points

1. Before proceeding to biopsy a full ENT examination should be performed to exclude a primary tumour of the head and neck. Sources of metastasis such as breast and gastrointestinal tract should also have been appropriately investigated.
2. Be careful to avoid any nerves that may lie in close proximity to the lymph node – especially the accessory and intercostobrachial.
3. A small piece of the lymph node should be sent for bacterial culture if TB is considered within the differential diagnosis.
4. Handle the specimen with care so as not to destroy the lymph node's architecture.
5. Do not biopsy lymph nodes in the neck under local anaesthesia.

RADICAL EXCISION OF TOE NAIL – ZADIK'S OPERATION

Indications

1. Ingrowing toenail not responding to conservative measures.
2. Onychogryphosis.
3. Chronic subungual infections.

Setting up

1. Local anaesthetic ring block.

Procedure

Perform a ring block using 3 ml of 1% lignocaine on each side. Introduce the needle vertically downwards, grazing the sides of the proximal phalanx. Aspirate the syringe each time before injecting and, if blood is seen, reposition the tip of the needle.

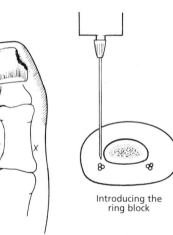

Injection sites

Introducing the ring block

Fig. 2.9

Apply a rubber tourniquet to the toe and, using a small-bladed scalpel, incise the nail bed and elevate flaps.

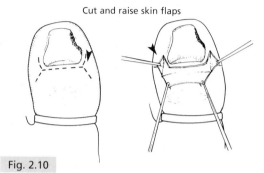

Cut and raise skin flaps

Fig. 2.10

Elevate the nail from its nail bed with a pair of heavy scissors and pull it off with a twisting motion.

Cut across the nail bed down to the bone and continue laterally as far as the nail fold. Remove the nail bed and place a single absorbable suture in the skin flaps on each side.

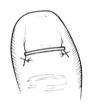

Fig. 2.11

Cover the toe with a simple dressing.

Key points

1. Never use adrenaline on the extremities.
2. If there is gross infection, treat with antibiotics and excise the nail at a later date.
3. Try and remove all the germinal matrix or a nail may regrow.
4. An alternative to excision is nail bed ablation with phenol. However, this is not advised for patients with diabetes or peripheral vascular disease or those on steroids.
5. If only part of the nail is troublesome a partial excision may be favourable.

3
HERNIAS

Indications

1. Inguinal hernia.
2. Patent processus vaginalis.

Setting up

1. General anaesthetic.
2. Supine position.

Procedure

Under general anaesthesia, make a 2 cm skin crease incision on the side of the hernia.

Pick up the skin edges with artery clips and deepen the incision to identify the cord under the external oblique. Divide the muscle along the length of its fibres.

Continue dissection down to the external ring. Free the cord posteriorly and pass a clip underneath the cord to allow some distal traction by the assistant.

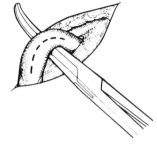

Fig. 3.2

This will allow easier dissection of the sac, which is positioned on the anterior and superior aspect of the cord. The dissection can be difficult. It is important to dissect the sac free posteriorly from the vas and vessels without damaging the sac if it extends down the cord.

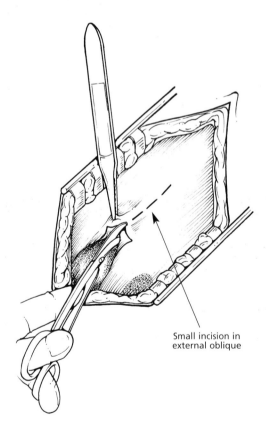

Small incision in external oblique

Fig. 3.1

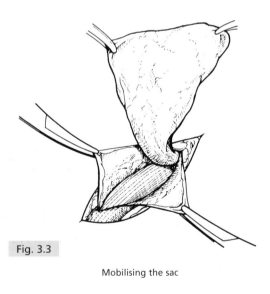

Fig. 3.3

Mobilising the sac

Patience and care are required. Open the sac to reduce its contents. This is particularly important in the female where an ovary may be present.

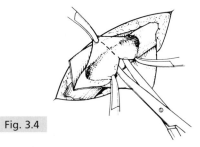

Fig. 3.4

Dividing across a thin-walled sac

Transfix the sac with an absorbable suture and excise the redundant tissue.

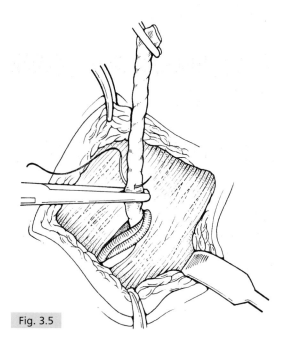

Fig. 3.5

Approximate the muscle with a couple of absorbable sutures and close the skin with an absorbable subcuticular suture.

Key points

1. Herniotomy is adequate in children.
2. Care in tissue handling is vital in order to prevent neurovascular damage.
3. Must ensure testis is in scrotum at the end of the procedure.
4. It is unnecessary to explore the contralateral groin 'just in case' there is an occult hernia. However, bilateral hernias in females should raise the possibility of intersex abnormalities.
5. Can usually safely be performed as day case.
6. The younger the child the more likely that the hernia will become obstructed or irreducible; therefore, young babies should be operated upon promptly.

Indications

Symptomatic hernias.

Setting up

1. General, local or regional anaesthesia.
2. Antibiotic prophylaxis if a synthetic non-absorbable mesh is used.
3. Supine position.

Procedure

After incising the skin 1 cm above and parallel to the inguinal ligament, incise the external oblique in the line of its fibres. Then, by pushing a dissecting scissors along the same line open the inguinal canal. Protect the ileoinguinal nerve if possible.

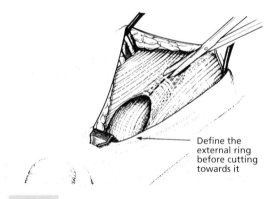

Define the external ring before cutting towards it

Fig. 3.6

Identify and retract the cord – a ring retractor helps.

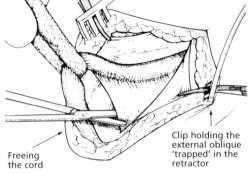

Freeing the cord

Clip holding the external oblique 'trapped' in the retractor

Fig. 3.7

Decide whether this is an indirect or a direct hernia by examining the posterior wall and dissecting any sac from the cord by sharp and blunt dissection.

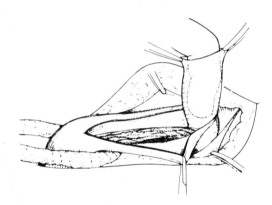

Fig. 3.8

Dissecting the sac wth a finger in it

Transfix and ligate the sac after having checked its contents (See Fig. 3.5).

There are now several options for the repair part of the procedure. The authors suggest that a polypropylene mesh repair is preferable in order to give a tension-free repair (Liechtenstein).

Take an 8 × 16 cm sheet of mesh and trim its ends to fit the medial end of the wound. Fix the mesh in place to the inguinal ligament using a non-absorbable continuous suture.

Medial   Lateral

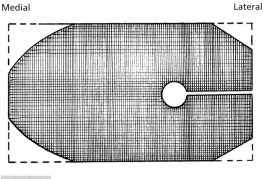

Fig. 3.9

Overlap the lateral borders around the cord and suture the lateral and superior borders of the mesh in place to the underlying muscle using interrupted non-absorbable sutures.

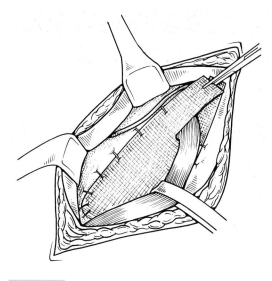

Fig. 3.10

Close the external oblique with a continuous absorbable suture and the skin with an absorbable subcuticular suture.

Key points

1. Most can be performed as day cases under local anaesthetic.
2. Technique is important in preventing complications and hernia recurrence.
3. In the case of an emergency presenting with obstruction, carefully examine the sac for the presence of bowel. If bowel is present it must be inspected. If the bowel is dusky in appearance wrap it in warm saline-soaked abdominal packs and leave it for a few minutes to see whether the appearance improves. If the bowel does not improve or if it appears necrotic it must be resected.
4. Must warn males, in particular those with recurrent hernias, of the possible need for orchidectomy.

Femoral hernia – all femoral hernias should be repaired.

Setting up

1. General anaesthetic is preferred, in particular for emergency cases in case necrotic bowel is found, but a local anaesthetic may be used.
2. Urinary catheter.
3. Supine position with 15° head-down tilt.

Procedure

There are three techniques for repair of a femoral hernia:

- Low or crural approach.
- High or inguinal approach.
- Extraperitoneal approach.

The inguinal approach is rarely adopted these days and will not be covered further.

Low approach

Make a small groin incision directly over the hernia, parallel to the inguinal ligament.

Identify and dissect the superficial fascia in the groin, down to the coverings of the hernia sac, and expose the neck of the hernia.

Sweep away the fascial coverings and open the hernial sac. Ligate and excise any redundant omentum and return any remaining tissue to the abdominal cavity. If you discover necrotic bowel perform a laparotomy. Transfix and ligate the sac at its neck and excise any redundant sac.

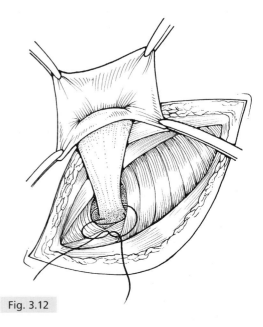

Fig. 3.12

Carefully retract the femoral vein and close the defect in the femoral canal. Use a non-absorbable suture on a J-shaped needle to approximate the lower border of the inguinal ligament to the fascia over pectineus muscle.

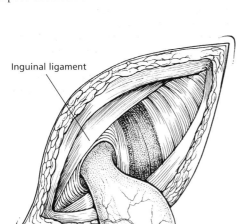

Inguinal ligament

Fig. 3.11

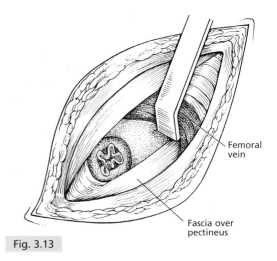

Femoral vein

Fascia over pectineus

Fig. 3.13

Close the subcutaneous tissues with interrupted absorbable sutures and the skin with a subcuticular suture.

Extraperitoneal approach

The hernia may be approached through a supra-inguinal, Pfannenstiel, midline or pararectal (McEvedy) incision.

Once through the skin, bluntly dissect the superficial tissues to gain access to the hernial sac. Open the rectus sheath and retract the rectus and open up the pre-peritoneal space with blunt dissection. Continue this process down towards the inguinal ligament and identify the hernia.

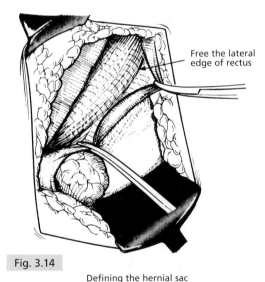

Free the lateral edge of rectus

Fig. 3.14

Defining the hernial sac

If the sac is empty reduce it back into the abdomen by pushing from below and gently pulling from above. If there is bowel present do not pull on the bowel but rather insert a haemostat and carefully stretch the femoral ring. Transfix the sac and excise any redundant tissue.

If the hernia cannot be reduced, open the peritoneum from above and inspect its contents. If the bowel appears of dubious viability an appropriate resection should be carried out.

Close the femoral canal with interrupted non-absorbable sutures between the pectineal ligament and the inguinal ligament.

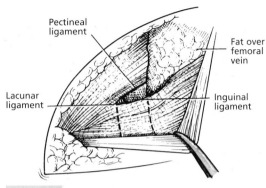

Pectineal ligament

Fat over femoral vein

Lacunar ligament

Inguinal ligament

Fig. 3.15

Closing the femoral canal from above

Close the rectus sheath with a non-absorbable suture and the skin with an absorbable subcuticular suture.

Key points

1. If you are not sure whether the hernia is an inguinal or femoral hernia use the extraperitoneal approach.
2. If there is any oozing from dissection of the sac, drain the area with a suction drain.
3. If there is any doubt about viability of bowel, having employed a low approach, a formal laparotomy is recommended to make sure that the bowel is not ischaemic.

UMBILICAL HERNIA REPAIR

Indications

1. Symptomatic umbilical hernias (rare).
2. Hernia still present at 4 years of age.

Setting up

1. General anaesthesia.
2. Supine position.

Procedure

Make a small stab incision transversely below the umbilicus and stretch it laterally by inserting the point of an artery forceps. Using this technique a neat curved incision is achieved.

Develop the plane using a mosquito clamp.

Identify the sac by passing a clip around the central defect.

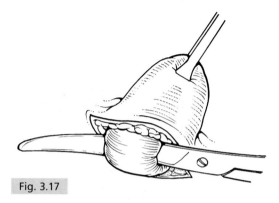

Fig. 3.17

Divide the sac from the umbilical skin and open the sac under direct vision, avoiding damage to underlying structures. Close the defect transversely using size 0 interrupted absorbable sutures. Double breasting of the defect is not required.

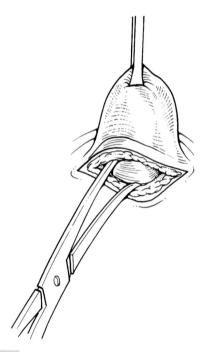

Fig. 3.16

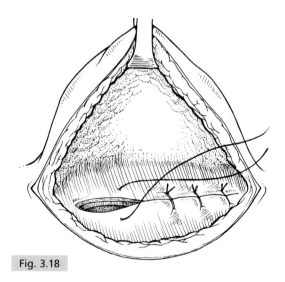

Fig. 3.18

It is important to tack the post-umbilical skin to the fascia to invert the umbilicus for cosmesis using absorbable sutures.

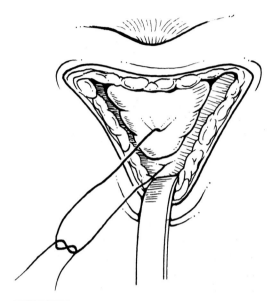

Fig. 3.19

Subcuticular closure of the skin is preferred.

Indications

1. Symptomatic including emergency.
2. Cosmetic.

Setting up

1. General or local anaesthetic.
2. Prophylactic antibiotics.
3. Anti-DVT (deep venous thrombosis) prophylaxis
   – stockings, minihep.
4. Supine position.

Procedure

Make a transverse incision encompassing the umbilicus and excise the ellipse of skin.

Further dissection may be rather bloody. It is important to identify and clear the aponeurotic edges of the defect prior to opening the sac and reducing its contents.

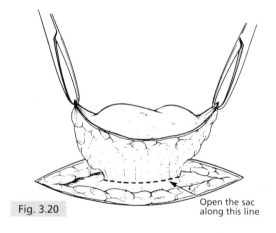

Fig. 3.20

Open the sac along this line

There may be many adhesions from the omentum and intestine to the sac, and care should be taken to free all these. Once the sac has been emptied excise the redundant sac and close the defect using a Mayo technique (or using interrupted non-absorbable mattress sutures).

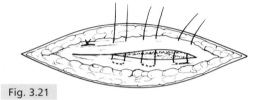

Fig. 3.21

Place all the overlapping sutures before tying them

If the subcutaneous defect is large, suction drainage should be employed. Close the skin with subcuticular absorbable sutures.

Key points

1. Ideally, all hernias should be repaired because of the risk of incarceration with omentum or intestine, which can be strangulated.
2. Encourage preoperative weight loss in the obese.
3. The incidence of infection is relatively high. Use antibiotic prophylaxis and meticulous haemostasis.
4. Patients sometimes develop postoperative 'ileus' if handling of the bowel is extensive.

Indications

All epigastric hernias should be repaired.

Setting up

1. General or local anaesthetic.
2. Supine position.

Procedure

If the diagnosis is certain and a single defect is present make a small transverse incision over the hernia. If, however, there is any doubt over the diagnosis or if there are multiple hernias choose a vertical incision.

Dissect the hernia from the surrounding abdominal wall, identify the defect in the linea alba and enlarge the defect transversely.

Incise the neck of the hernia, inspect its contents and return them to the peritoneal cavity, usually extraperitoneal fat.

If a sac is present, transfix its neck with an absorbable suture and excise the redundant sac. Repair the defect in the linea alba with interrupted non-absorbable sutures. Place all sutures first before tying them.

Close the skin with subcuticular absorbable sutures.

Key points

1. Patients with epigastric hernias often report severe abdominal pain due to strangulation of the extraperitoneal sac. Others report chronic epigastric discomfort; in this case peptic ulcer disease and gallstones must be excluded.
2. Make sure the site is marked preoperatively as epigastric hernias can be difficult to find when the patient is anaesthetised.

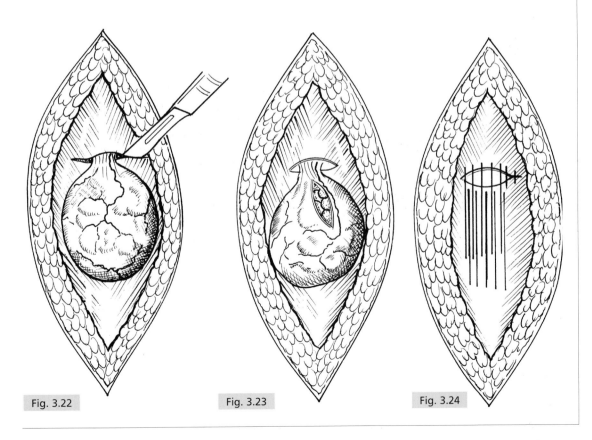

Fig. 3.22   Fig. 3.23   Fig. 3.24

Indications

1. Symptomatic.
2. Cosmetic.

Setting up

1. General anaesthetic.
2. Prophylactic antibiotics.
3. Anti-DVT prophylaxis – stockings, minihep.
4. Supine position.

Procedure

Approach the defect by making an elliptical incision to include the previous scar.

Excise the scar, taking care not to take too much skin as this will create undue tension at the time of wound closure.

Dissect the hernia from the surrounding subcutaneous tissues. Proceed laterally so as to allow exposure of healthy tissue all around the hernia.

Define the sac and dissect down to the neck of the hernia. Fully identify the aponeurotic defect. Open the hernia sac and examine its contents.

If the contents are viable, divide any adhesions that may exist with the hernia sac and return them to the peritoneal cavity. If the hernia is strangulated perform an appropriate resection at this time. Excise the redundant sac and close the opening in the peritoneum with a continuous absorbable suture.

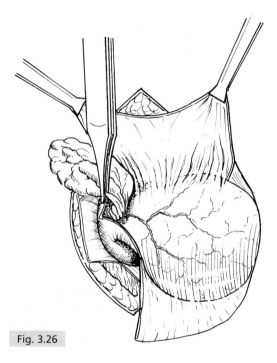

Fig. 3.26

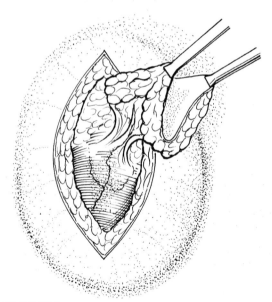

Fig. 3.25

It is important to dissect healthy aponeurotic tissue on each side of the defect. Insert a suction drain and close the aponeurotic layer with interrupted double near-and-far nylon sutures. Insert all sutures before tying them.

Reinforce this repair with an overlay of mesh and secure this in place with interrupted non-absorbable sutures.

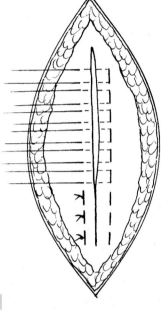

Fig. 3.27

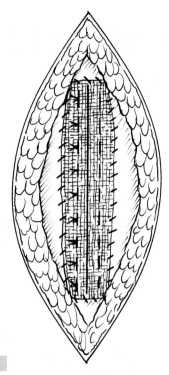

Fig. 3.28

Close the skin with subcuticular absorbable sutures.

Key points

1. Incisional hernias usually occur as a result of poor surgical technique at the initial wound closure, and so to prevent incisional hernias the most important lesson is to close the wound satisfactorily the first time around.
2. If the hernia is large with a complex defect, computed tomography may help to delineate the lesion.
3. Incisional hernias can be difficult. An experienced surgeon is the most important factor in preventing recurrence!

4

BREAST

Indications

1. Benign, e.g. fibroadenoma.
2. Possibly malignant lump, e.g. equivocal triple assessment (clinical/mammography/cytology).

Setting up

1. Local or general anaesthetic.

Procedure

Fix the position of the lump between finger and thumb before commencing, as many lumps 'disappear' once the skin is incised. If you still have difficulty, dip your fingers in skin preparation fluid (e.g. Savlon) and try again. The incision can be placed circumferentially if close to the nipple, or radially if placed distally.

Grasp the lump with a pair of tissue forceps and retract it out of the wound as the surrounding tissue is divided with a knife.

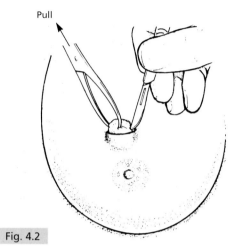

Pull

Fig. 4.2

Use a pair of Langenbeck retractors to expose the interior of the cavity and diathermy all bleeding points. Obliterate the cavity with interrupted absorbable sutures, taking care not to distort the symmetry of the breasts. Large wounds should be drained with a suction drain. The skin should be closed with a subcuticular absorbable suture.

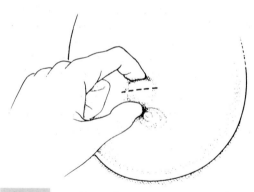

Fig. 4.1

Fix the lump as you cut

Key points

1. Haematomas may be a significant problem if haemostasis is not ensured, as they may hinder further imaging of the breast or may become secondarily infected.

Indications

1. Radiographically identified microcalcification suspicious of ductal carcinoma in situ.
2. Impalpable lesion suspicious of carcinoma.

The localisation process may be performed using either ultrasound or X-rays and is usually performed by a radiologist. The guide-wire is barbed so as to hold its position in the breast. Mammograms confirming the correct placement of the wire are taken to theatre with the patient.

Setting up

1. General anaesthetic.
2. Take care to prepare the whole length of the exposed wire with antiseptic solution.

Procedure

Using the mammograms to predict the course of the wire, determine the most suitable point for the incision and incise the skin transversely.

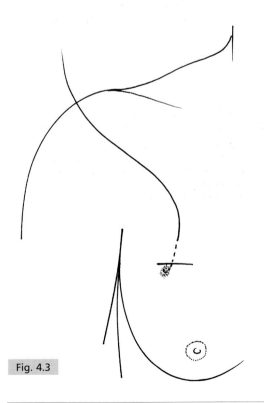

Fig. 4.3

Locate the wire and pull the distal end through the skin into the wound.

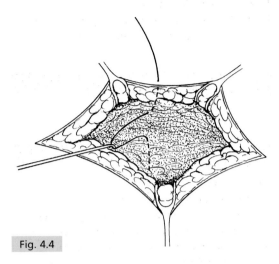

Fig. 4.4

Follow the wire into the substance of the breast, taking care not to displace the wire. Excise around the wire with a good clearance margin. Mark the specimen with sutures so as to allow orientation by the pathologist. Whilst the patient is anaesthetised send the specimen for radiological assessment. If the lesion is not present or is incompletely excised further excision of the cavity may be performed.

When the adequacy of the excision has been confirmed, ensure meticulous haemostasis. Close the cavity with interrupted absorbable sutures and a subcuticular absorbable suture for the skin.

Key points

1. Take care not to disturb the position of the wire during transport of the patient.

WIDE LOCAL EXCISION AND AXILLARY CLEARANCE

Indications

Tumours of 4 cm or less with positive triple assessment and a mammogram that excludes multifocal disease.

Setting up

1. General anaesthesia.
2. Anti-DVT prophylaxis – stockings, minihep.
3. Position supine with arm on arm board. Occlusive stockinette dressings are applied so as to allow manoeuvre of the arm peroperatively.

Procedure

Mark out a curvilinear incision preoperatively, ensuring that a cosmetically acceptable closure is possible. When deciding on the size of the incision ensure that you have included any previous biopsy sites within your margins.

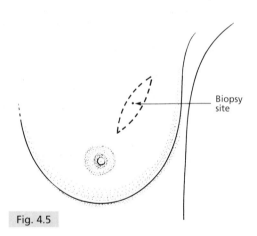

Biopsy site

Fig. 4.5

Incise around the segment and deepen the incision, keeping well away from the tumour (at least 1 cm clearance). This is best accomplished with diathermy. When the pectoralis fascia is encountered, separate the breast tissue from the fascia and remove the tumour, taking care to maintain its orientation. Insert silk sutures using a recognisable coding system in order to identify superior, inferior, medial, lateral, superficial and deep margins of the specimen.

Coagulate any bleeding points with diathermy. One or two suction drains may be required, depending upon the amount of bleeding encountered. Wash the wound with antiseptic solution and then place a couple of interrupted absorbable sutures in the subcutaneous tissues to maintain tissue alignment. Skin closure may be with suture or staples.

It is important to perform a full dissection of the axillary lymph nodes in order to correctly stage the tumour and thus provide prognostic information. This consists of excision of all lymph nodes up to the medial border of pectoralis minor (Level II).

The axilla should be approached through a separate laterally placed incision.

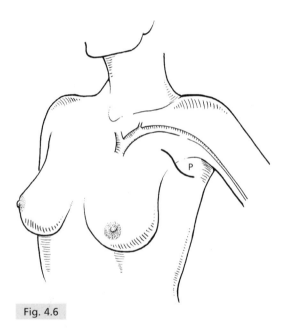

P

Fig. 4.6

Elevate the skin flaps superiorly and inferiorly. Using a combination of blunt and sharp dissection, identify the lateral border of pectoralis major and the anterior border of latissimus dorsi which form the anterior and posterior borders for the dissection.

Identify and divide pectoralis minor, allowing access to the Level II nodes. Identify and preserve the thoracodorsal and long thoracic nerves. The intercostobrachial nerve is often encountered and should be preserved if possible.

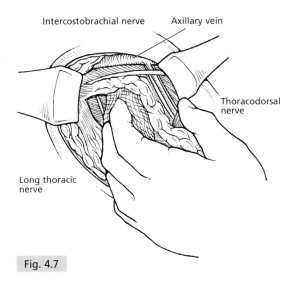

Fig. 4.7

The upper limit for dissection is the axillary vein. Dissect the axillary tissue from the vein using a Lahey swab, taking care to ligate the venous tributaries as they are encountered.

Gently dissect the axillary contents away from the nerves and their companion arteries using a gauze swab. The axillary contents can now be removed *en bloc*. Drain the axilla with a suction drain. Wash the wound with antiseptic betadine and then close the subcutaneous tissues with interrupted absorbable sutures followed by a subcuticular suture for the skin.

Apply a light dressing to the wound and cover it with strips of Elastoplast to apply pressure to the wound. The pressure dressing is removed after 24 hours.

Key points

1. Haematomas can be avoided provided you follow the above steps, namely diathermy, drains, deep stitches and pressure dressings.
2. Informed consent should include mention of axillary numbness after surgery due to trauma/sacrifice of the intercostobrachial nerve.
3. Make sure that the axillary dissection is carried out correctly and not a 'sampling' procedure since the combination of axillary surgery and radiotherapy has a high risk for the development of lymphoedema.
4. In order to provide a good cosmetic result the breast must be of adequate size and shape.

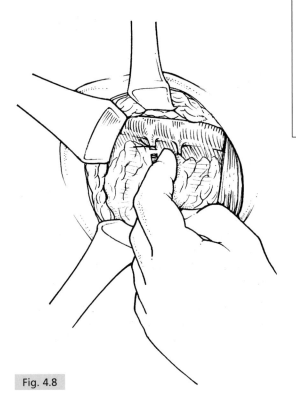

Fig. 4.8

Indications

Cytolologically proven breast carcinoma.

Setting up

1. General anaesthesia.
2. Anti-DVT prophylaxis – stockings, minihep.
3. Position supine with arm on arm board. Occlusive stockinette dressings are applied so as to allow manoeuvre of the arm preoperatively.

Procedure

Mark the boundaries for the skin incision prior to commencing the operation. These should be at least 3 cm from the tumour. The anatomical markers for the operation are delineated medially by the sternum, laterally by latissimus dorsi, superiorly by the clavicle and inferiorly a point 1–2 cm below the inframammary fold.

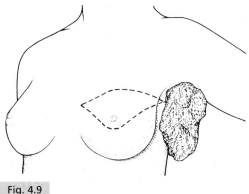

Fig. 4.9

Incise along the skin incisions with a knife and then dissect the skin flaps from the breast tissue below. Start with the upper flap. Place three pairs of tissue forceps on the subcuticular tissue of the skin margin for your assistant to apply traction, and apply caudally directed counter-traction to the breast tissue. Dissection should be carried out aiming for a thickness of 3–4 mm medially and increasing to about 6–8 mm laterally.

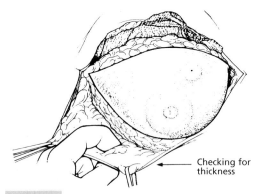

Checking for thickness

Fig. 4.10

As the inferior border of the clavicle is encountered begin dissecting more deeply until the fascia overlying pectoralis major is visible. This dissection may be performed with either a knife or diathermy.

Bleeding from perforating vessels is commonly encountered as the dissection approaches the sternum and must be rapidly controlled with coagulative diathermy or ligation. The inferior flap is raised in a similar manner.

Having attained haemostasis of the breast base turn your attention to the axilla. Peel the breast laterally until the anterior border of latissimus dorsi is reached. Pectoralis major is retracted medially to expose pectoralis minor. This in turn is retracted medially and anteriorly. A finger is then passed underneath the muscle and the muscle is divided close to its point of insertion onto the coracoid process of the scapula.

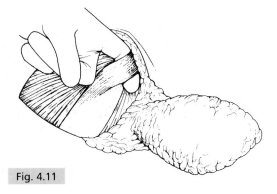

Fig. 4.11

Commencing caudal to the axillary vein, dissection is carried out only after identification of the long thoracic and thoracodorsal nerves. Use a Lahey swab to gently sweep the axillary contents from the axillary vein and ligate all venous tributaries.

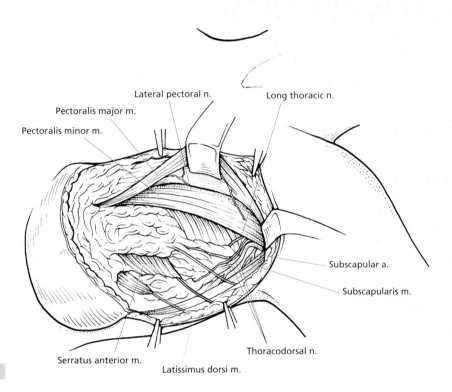

Pectoralis major m.
Pectoralis minor m.
Lateral pectoral n.
Long thoracic n.
Subscapular a.
Subscapularis m.
Serratus anterior m.
Latissimus dorsi m.
Thoracodorsal n.

Fig. 4.12

The axillary contents are removed in continuity with the breast, having labelled the most proximal lymph node with a stitch for pathological orientation of the specimen.

Place one suction drain on the breast bed and one in the axilla. Wash out the wound with antiseptic betadine prior to closing. The subcutaneous tissues are approximated with interrupted absorbable sutures and the skin closed with a subcuticular suture or staples. A lightweight dressing should be applied to the wound and secured with adhesive tape so as to apply pressure to the wound.

Key points

1. Haemostasis is of crucial importance. It is worth spending an extra few minutes at the time of surgery rather than having to bring the patient back to theatre or dealing with an infected haematoma.
2. Take care not to dissect the skin flaps too thinly or they might buttonhole.
3. Identification of the long thoracic is crucial in order to prevent winging of the scapula; also the thoracodorsal nerve must be identified and preserved so as not to cause motor loss to latissimus dorsi.
4. If you encounter excess tension on trying to close the skin, you should further undermine the skin flaps, as closing under tension may lead to flap necrosis. If there is still inadequate coverage consider a split-skin graft.
5. The option of immediate reconstruction should be discussed with the patient before the operation.

Gynaecomastia.

Setting up

1. General anaesthetic.

Procedure

Make a curved incision in the submammary skin.

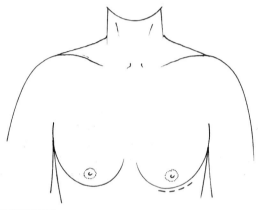

Fig. 4.13

Raise a superior flap by dissecting between the skin and the breast tissue. As the nipple is approached make a point of cutting at an angle of 45° to include most of the ductal tissue.

Cut down (at 45°) as you go under the nipple

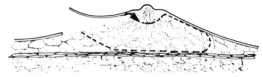

Fig. 4.14

Having completed excision of the ducts return to dissection in the subcutaneous plane above the nipple. When all the skin has been dissected off the breast mound, dissect downwards until the deep fascia overlying pectoralis major is encountered. The breast tissue can now be removed.

Insert Langenbeck retractors to inspect the cavity and allow control of bleeding with diathermy. Introduce a suction drain and close the skin. Apply a pressure dressing to the wound.

Key points

1. Breast tissue is not always easy to distinguish from subcutaneous fat, so don't take too much.
2. It is good practice to leave a little duct tissue beneath the nipple so as to avoid a disfiguring appearance.
3. Don't worry about the initial postoperative appearance as considerable remodelling occurs over the subsequent months.
4. For large gynaecomastia a combination of excision and liposuction may be more appropriate.

Indications

Persistent blood-stained discharge from a single duct opening on the nipple.

Setting up

1. General or local anaesthesia.

Procedure

Squeeze the breast and nipple area until a drop of discharge is seen.

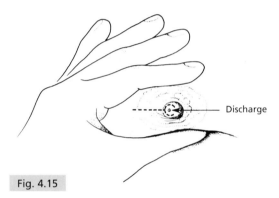

— Discharge

Fig. 4.15

Cannulate the duct opening using a lacrimal probe and secure the probe in place using a size 3/0 suture that has been passed through the skin alongside the duct opening. Make a radial incision into the skin of the nipple along the line of the probe, encircling the duct orifice.

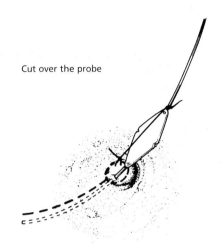

Cut over the probe

Fig. 4.16

Dissect the skin of the areola away from the underlying breast tissue for approximately 1 cm on each side of the probe and excise the breast segment containing the probe with the aid of scissors, commencing behind the duct orifice and continuing into the breast.

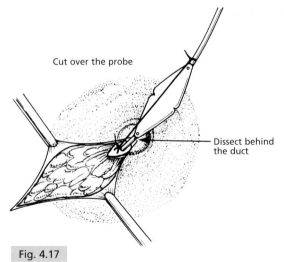

Cut over the probe

— Dissect behind the duct

Fig. 4.17

Secure haemostasis with diathermy and approximate the breast tissue with interrupted absorbable sutures. Close the skin incision with a subcuticular absorbable suture.

Key points

1. Leaving a transparent adhesive dressing over the nipple for 24 hours prior to surgery will help localise the discharge.
2. Do not be too forceful with the probe as this may cause a false passage.
3. A pressure dressing will help to prevent haematoma formation.

Indications

1. Blood-stained or serous discharge from one or more ducts in women aged over 40 years.
2. Duct ectasia with discharge sufficient to embarrass or inconvenience the patient.

Setting up

1. General anaesthetic.

Procedure

Approach the ducts through a periareolar incision as it provides both good access and good cosmesis.

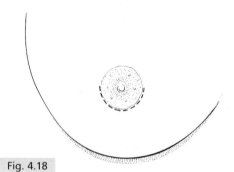

Fig. 4.18

Deepen the incision through the subcutaneous tissues, taking care to ligate all vessels with absorbable sutures. The correct plane for dissection lies between the fat lobules of the breast and the areola, thus preserving the subdermal vascular plexus. Elevate the areola with hooks to expose the main ductal system, then pass a curved artery forceps behind the nipple so as to create a tunnel.

Key points

1. Take care not to extend the incision beyond 180° as this increases the risk of nipple necrosis.

Grasp the ductal tissue and cut it close to the under-surface of the nipple.

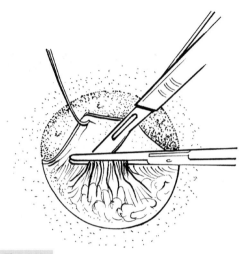

Fig. 4.19

Deal immediately with bleeding vessels before they retract. Examine for completeness of excision by inverting the nipple and trimming any residual duct with scissors.

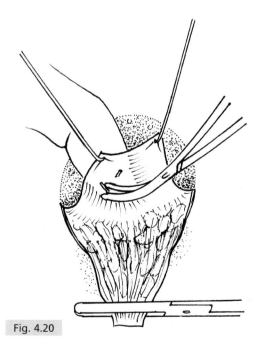

Fig. 4.20

Close the skin with interrupted size 4/0 absorbable sutures. A suction drain may be required.

Indications

Breast abscess.

Setting up

1. General anaesthetic.
2. Intravenous antibiotics on induction.
3. Supine position.

Procedure

Identify the most fluctuant part of the abscess. Centre a radial incision over the abscess and incise into the abscess cavity. Have a pus swab at the ready and obtain a good sample of pus and send it for culture and sensitivity studies.

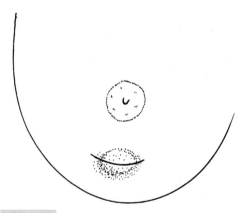

Fig. 4.21

Insert a finger into the cavity and ensure that all loculations are adequately broken down.

The abscess cavity may be filled with an alginate dressing or a corrugated drain may be left in situ.

If the cavity is very large a second incision may be made to allow dependent drainage of pus. In this case the drain may be led through one incision and out through the other.

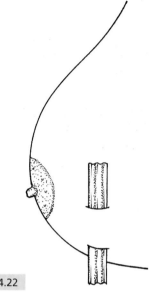

Fig. 4.22

Cover the wound with an absorbent dressing and provide support with a well-fitting bra.

Key points

1. If an abscess has evidence of tissue destruction, e.g. skin ischaemia, proceed to early drainage as failure to do so may lead to a permanent deformity.
2. It is worth taking a biopsy in all cases so as not to be caught out by an inflammatory carcinoma.
3. If the patient has systemic signs of sepsis or associated cellulitis the antibiotics should be continued postoperatively.
4. Repeated aspiration or percutaneous drainage under ultrasound now successfully treats many breast abscesses.

5

UPPER GASTROINTESTINAL

Indications

Diagnostic

Evaluation of upper gastrointestinal symptoms.

Therapeutic

1. Injection of bleeding varices/ulcers.
2. Insertion of feeding tubes, e.g. percutaneous endoscopic gastrostomy (PEG) p. 50.
3. Insertion of luminal stents.
4. Dilatation of oesophageal strictures.

Setting up

1. Procedure usually performed under intravenous sedation or topical anaesthesia to the oropharynx.
2. Constant monitoring of oxygen saturation.
3. Position in left lateral decubitus position, facing the surgeon.

Procedure

Prior to starting, it is important to familiarise oneself with the controls of the instrument, including directional control of the tip as well as washing and aspiration facilities.

Place a mouthguard so as to protect the endoscope. Insert the scope under direct vision taking care to stay in the midline. Ask the patient to swallow when they feel pressure from the scope.

The oesophagus

Advance the scope slowly, keeping the instrument central. Insufflate with air as required in order to adequately distend the oesophagus for inspection. It is important to inspect the whole circumference thoroughly to exclude a mucosal lesion.

The first landmark is the extraluminal compression caused by the left main bronchus and aortic arch. The gastro-oesophageal junction lies at 38–40 cm and is characterised by a change in colour and a serrated appearance due to a change in mucosa. The level of the oesophageal hiatus can be established by asking the patient to inspire deeply as this causes the hiatus to indent the oesophageal wall.

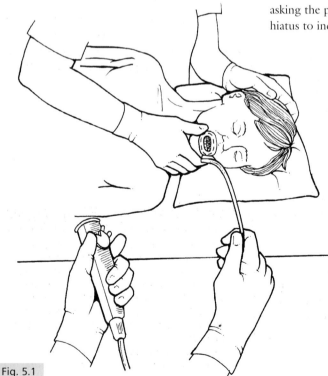

Fig. 5.1

The stomach

Rotating the tip around the axis of the endoscope as it is advanced into the stomach allows visualisation of the anterior and posterior walls as well as most of the lesser and greater curvatures of the stomach.

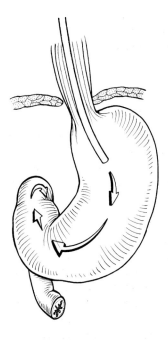

Fig. 5.2

Further advance the scope towards the prepyloric area. Identify the pylorus and position the scope just above the pylorus. When the pylorus relaxes advance the scope into the duodenum and perform a thorough inspection of the mucosa.

After completing examination of the duodenum, draw back the scope through the pylorus. Perform a 'J' manoeuvre in order to visualise the cardia, fundus and upper parts of both greater and lesser curves. In order to do this, rotate the scope towards the greater curvature and then angulate the tip upward 180°.

Slowly withdraw the scope whilst rotating the tip so as to allow visualisation of proximal structures. You can be sure that you have completed the manoeuvre when you visualise the endoscope entering the stomach.

At the end of the inspection straighten the scope prior to withdrawing it into the oesophagus. The large volume of air insufflated to allow visualisation causes patient discomfort and nausea so it is important to remove all the air before withdrawing the scope at the end of the procedure.

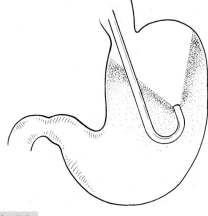

Fig. 5.3

Obtaining tissue specimens

Mucosal lesions identified during endoscopy can be biopsied using a cup forceps that is introduced through a side port of the scope. The biopsies may be subjected to histological examination or placed in culture media for *H. pylori*.

Key points

1. Patient monitoring is vitally important, in particular when sedation is administered.
2. A slow and cautious advancement of the scope with careful inspection of the entire mucosal surface of the oesophagus and stomach is critical. Rough handling may lead to mucosal trauma and bleeding which prevents complete visualisation.
3. It is important to adequately biopsy all suspicious lesions at several sites.

Indications

Long-term enteral nutrition when oral ingestion is not possible, e.g following cerebrovascular accident.

Setting up

1. Local anaesthesia to the skin and topical anaesthesia to the oropharynx.

Procedure

The optimal site for the gastrostomy is usually indicated by a point one-third of the way from the rib margin (at the mid-clavicular line) to the umbilicus.

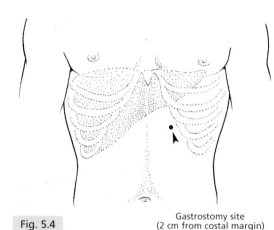

Fig. 5.4

Gastrostomy site
(2 cm from costal margin)

Insert a gastroscope and insufflate air in order to distend the stomach. Carry out a full endoscopic examination of the stomach. Indent the abdominal wall with a finger over the proposed gastrostomy site. If there are no interposing organs a clear indentation will be seen through the endoscope. If this view is not clear, the transverse colon may be obstructing the planned course of the gastrostomy. An alternative method to confirm a suitable

position is to switch off the theatre lights and observe for clear light from the scope.

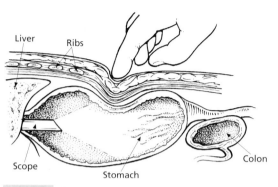

Liver   Ribs

Scope   Stomach   Colon

Fig. 5.5

Make a small incision in the skin of the abdominal wall and insert the trocar needle under direct vision into the stomach. Pass the nylon loop through the trocar and then grasp the loop with a snare or biopsy forceps passed through the gastroscope.

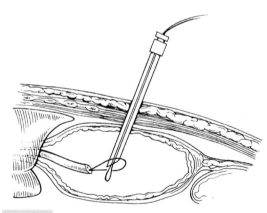

Fig. 5.6

Withdraw the gastroscope and snare, drawing the nylon loop through the mouth.

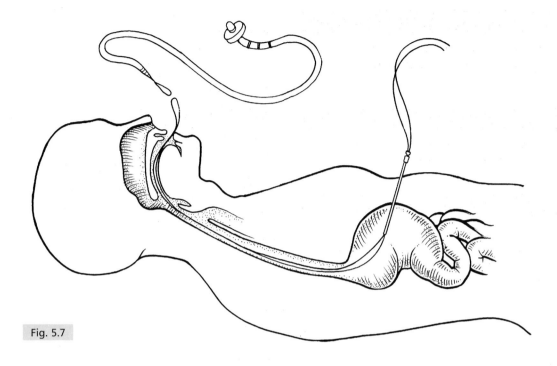

Fig. 5.7

Tie the gastrostomy tube to the nylon loop, drawing it back into the stomach and then out through the abdominal wall. Pass the retaining disc over the gastrostomy tube in order to fix it in position.

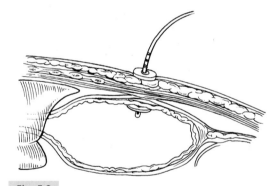

Fig. 5.8

Key points

1. If you are unsure as to whether there may be a viscus between stomach and abdominal wall then choose an alternative position for the gastrostomy.
2. Keep the discs tightly opposed for 48 hours so as to prevent the gastrostomy from migrating.
3. Leave the gastrostomy to drain for 24 hours and then commence feeding.
4. A post-procedure endoscopy is not required.

Indications

1. Pyloric stenosis due to scarring or tumour.
2. As an alternative to pyloroplasty following vagotomy.

Setting up

1. General anaesthetic.
2. Nasogastric tube.
3. Antibiotic prophylaxis.
4. Anti-DVT prophylaxis – stockings, minihep.
5. Urinary catheter.
6. Supine position.

Procedure

Anterior gastroenterostomy

Through an upper midline incision lift up the transverse mesocolon and identify the proximal jejunum as it commences at the ligament of Treitz. Bring a loop of the proximal jejunum around the transverse colon and the greater omentum so that it lies comfortably alongside the anterior wall of the stomach. Construct a side-to-side anastomosis, starting with a continuous seromuscular suture between the stomach and jejunum using an absorbable suture.

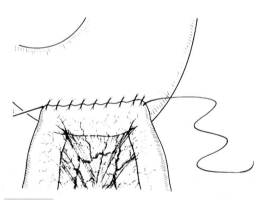

Fig. 5.9

Posterior seromuscular suture

Using a cutting diathermy, make a 5 cm incision in the jejunum, keeping just to one side of the row of sutures, then perform a similar-length incision on the stomach.

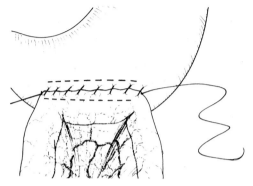

Fig. 5.10

Take full-thickness bites of stomach and jejunum

Using a double-ended absorbable suture, place the first stitch through the full-thickness of the posterior wall of the stomach and jejunum at the midpoint of the anastomosis. Tie the suture so that both ends are equal, then continue the posterior-wall anastomosis using a full-thickness over-and-over technique until you reach the corner.

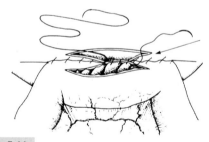

Fig. 5.11

Perform the same procedure in the opposite direction until the corner is reached. For the corners, continue in the same fashion, i.e. inside out, outside in.

Continue the anastomosis of the anterior aspect using a full-thickness continuous suture until the two lengths of suture meet in the midline. Having tied the suture, the anterior anastomosis is completed by inserting a continuous seromuscular suture. The same suture used for the posterior seromuscular suture can be used for this, and when completed it is tied to its own end.

A drain is not usually required. Close the wound as for a midline laparotomy.

Posterior gastroenterostomy

Detach the greater omentum from the greater curve of the stomach over a distance of 10 cm to allow access to the lesser sac. Lift up the transverse colon and make a 7 cm window in the base of the mesocolon to the left of the middle colic vessels, and where there are no obvious vessels crossing. Identify the loop of jejunum as for the anterior gastroenterostomy and pass a loop of bowel through the window so that it lies within the lesser sac. Apply a non-crushing forceps to the proximal limb of the jejunum as a marker and take care that the jejunum has not twisted during manipulation. Perform an anastomosis between the stomach and jejunum, using the same technique as for the anterior approach.

Having completed the anastomosis, lift up the transverse colon and pull the jejunal loop back through the mesocolon until the anastomosis becomes visible. Place a few interrupted absorbable sutures between the edge of the mesocolon and the stomach.

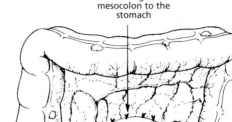

Tack the edge of the mesocolon to the stomach

Fig. 5.13

A drain is not usually required. Close the wound as for a midline laparotomy.

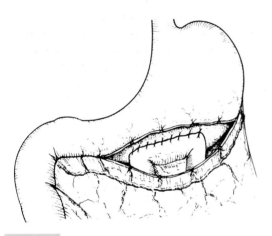

Fig. 5.12

Posterior gastrojejunostomy

Key points

1. The anterior approach is the simpler option; however, it is less physiological than the posterior gastroenterostomy and is more prone to obstruction.
2. Check very carefully the segment of bowel being used and ensure that it is not twisted.
3. The gastroenterostomy should be isoperistaltic in that the peristalsis in the apex of the loop should be from right to left.
4. Ensure good haemostasis, particularly on the gastric side of the anastomosis.

Indications

Acute duodenal perforation.

Setting up

1. General anaesthetic.
2. Nasogastric tube.
3. Antibiotic prophylaxis.
4. Anti-DVT prophylaxis – stockings, minihep.
5. Urinary catheter.
6. Supine position.

Procedure

Through an upper midline laparotomy identify the stomach and work distally to the duodenum. Perforations are usually found on the anterior surface of the first part of the duodenum.

Identify the perforation and insert three absorbable sutures through the duodenum on each side of the perforation.

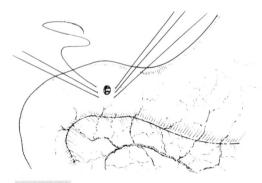

Fig. 5.14

Find a piece of omentum that can easily be mobilised into position, lay it across the perforation and loosely tie the sutures over the top of the omentum.

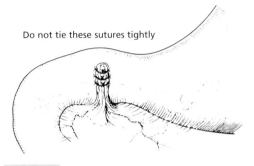

Do not tie these sutures tightly

Fig. 5.15

Wash out the peritoneal cavity thoroughly to remove food residue and close as for a laparotomy.

Key points

1. Do not tie the omentum too tightly or it may necrose.
2. If no perforation is evident on the anterior surface, mobilise the posterior surface of the stomach. If a perforated gastric ulcer is found take several biopsies as it may be malignant. If the perforation is small close it in the same way as for a duodenal ulcer. If the ulcer is large and friable a partial gastrectomy is required.

Indications

Bleeding from an ulcer that has failed to respond to conservative management or endoscopic therapy.

Setting up

1. General anaesthetic.
2. Nasogastric tube.
3. Antibiotic prophylaxis.
4. Anti-DVT prophylaxis – stockings, minihep.
5. Urinary catheter.
6. Supine position.

Procedure

After opening the abdomen through a midline incision, you will find the stomach distended with blood and the small bowel will appear grey due to the presence of blood within its lumen. Insert two stay sutures in the duodenal wall and open the duodenum longitudinally.

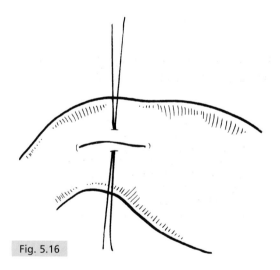

Fig. 5.16

Pass a sucker into the duodenal lumen to identify the bleeding point of the ulcer, which is usually seen on the posterior wall. It may be useful to stuff a swab into the pylorus to prevent blood being expelled from the stomach from obstructing the view. Under-run the gastroduodenal artery as it passes behind the duodenum using a size 1 absorbable suture.

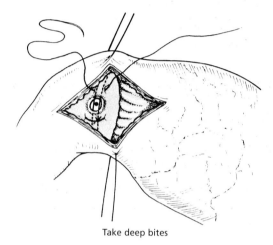

Take deep bites

Fig. 5.17

Take good-sized bites or you will miss the artery altogether but don't go too deep as the common bile duct lies in close proximity. Tie the sutures firmly and make sure the bleeding has ceased. Remove the gauze swab and then evacuate the blood clot from the stomach. Depending upon the degree of ulcer-related duodenal scarring proceed to a pyloroplasty or gastroenterostomy.

A drain is not usually required. Close the wound as for a midline laparotomy.

Key points

1. If you cannot identify a source in the duodenum, suspect a source in the stomach. Extend the incision proximally to look for missed pathology such as gastric ulcer, erosions or varices.

Indications

1. Symptomatic gallstones causing cholecystitis, biliary colic or pancreatitis.
2. Mucocele or empyema of gallbladder.
3. Acalculous cholecystitis.

Setting up

1. General anaesthetic.
2. Nasogastric tube.
3. Antibiotic prophylaxis.
4. Anti-DVT prophylaxis – stockings, minihep.
5. Urinary catheter or recent micturltion documented.
6. Position supine on X-ray table with image intensifier available. If screening facilities are not available it is important that the patient is correctly placed with the tip of the ninth rib over the middle of the cassette and the iliac crest on the edge of the film (Fig. 5.18).
7. Instrument check – make sure instruments are in good working order including: Verres needle is sharp with good spring, functioning suction/irrigation device.

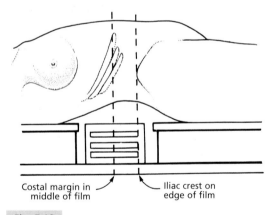

Costal margin in middle of film   Iliac crest on edge of film

Fig. 5.18

Procedure

Place the patient in a reverse Trendelenburg position in order to move small intestine away from pelvis. Set up as for laparoscopy and insert an umbilical trocar.

Place the remaining trocars as shown.

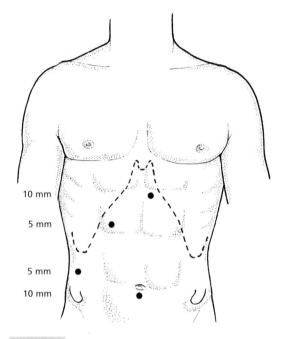

10 mm

5 mm

5 mm

10 mm

Fig. 5.19

Insert the 10 mm epigastric trocar under direct vision, just to the right of the midline opposite the middle of the costal margin. It is often beneficial to place the trocar to the right of the falciform ligament to facilitate instrument access. Place the two 5 mm cannulae in the right anterior axillary line and the mid-clavicular line again under direct vision. These positions can vary depending on patient anatomy. A fifth port may be necessary in obese individuals or in those with a Riedel's lobe. Now move the patient into a Trendelenburg position with left lateral roll to move omentum from right upper quadrant.

Grasp the gallbladder with the lateral 5 mm instrument and retract cranially. Use the second 5 mm grasper to hold the body of the gallbladder during dissection.

Using a 5 mm dissecting forceps, e.g. Petelin or Maryland, peel the peritoneum overlying the fundus of the gallbladder extending dissection over the cystic duct into Calot's triangle. Dissect the cystic duct, using the mid-clavicular grasper to lift the gallbladder cranially in order to develop a window for dissection.

the cystic duct and insert the cannula. Stabilise the cannula by the application of light pressure using a clip applicator. Raise the left side of the table by 10–15 degrees so that the biliary tree does not overlap the lumbar spine. Image intensification is preferred because the ports can often obscure the anatomy and can be moved by the operator.

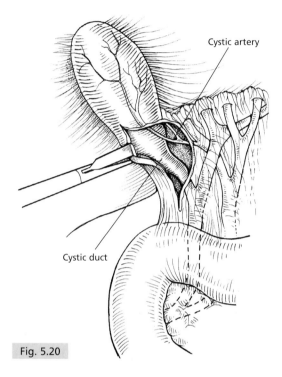

Cystic artery

Cystic duct

Fig. 5.20

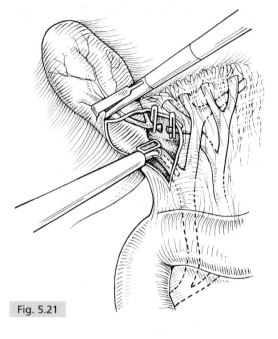

Fig. 5.21

Do not divide, clip or diathermy any structure until the anatomy is clearly visible. Do not dissect the junction of the cystic duct and common bile duct. Blunt dissection will nearly always be adequate and diathermy should be avoided if possible at this stage (see section on diathermy in Chapter 1).

If stones are present consider the alternatives: carrying on with laparoscopic cholecystectomy with a view to early ERCP, laparoscopic exploration of the bile duct, or conversion to open cholecystectomy. This is controversial.

Operative cholangiography

There is controversy regarding the performance of routine cholangiography. However, in situations where the anatomy is unclear, facilities must be available and a safe and consistent technique is therefore required.

Having clipped the gallbladder fundus and cystic artery, introduce a long needle trocar with a cannula under direct vision. Make a small incision in

Having completed cholangiography, clip and divide the cystic duct.

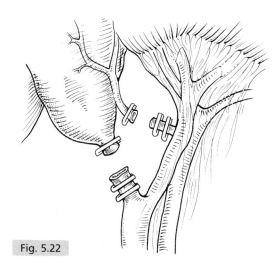

Fig. 5.22

The golden rule is that dissection must be as close to the gallbladder as possible to avoid any danger with aberrant anatomy.

The gallbladder is now free for dissection from the liver bed. This can be accomplished by sharp and blunt dissection or by diathermy or by ultrasonic water dissection. Stay close to the gallbladder to avoid excess bleeding from the liver.

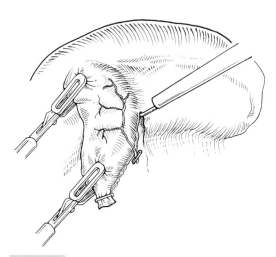

Fig. 5.23

Use the suction/irrigation device to maintain good visibility.

If you pierce the gallbladder and stones are spilled, try to retrieve them. It may be necessary to introduce a disposable bag to place stones and gallbladder in to minimise spillage.

Use irrigation with heparinised saline to facilitate clot removal. The gallbladder can be removed via either the umbilical or epigastric ports. Removal via the epigastric port does not entail any loss or disorientation of the visual image. A drain can be introduced via either of the 5 mm ports and can be placed directly into the liver bed.

Key points

1. Patients with a high risk of common duct stones should be identified in advance of laparoscopic cholecystectomy and undergo ERCP initially.
2. Laparoscopic cholecystectomy is best avoided in patients on anticoagulants.
3. Laparoscopic cholecystectomy is best avoided if the ultrasound is suspicious of gallbladder malignancy.
4. If the gallbladder is tense and distended it should be decompressed to aid grasping.
5. There are a number of important anatomical variations of both the arterial supply and biliary drainage so be very careful to identify all structures correctly before dividing them. If at any time there is doubt about anatomy or complications of bleeding call for assistance and have a low threshold for conversion to open procedure.

Indications

1. As for laparoscopic cholecystectomy.
2. The presence of a contraindication to laparoscopic cholecystectomy.
3. Failed laparoscopic procedure.

Setting up

1. General anaesthetic.
2. Nasogastric tube.
3. Antibiotic prophylaxis.
4. Anti-DVT prophylaxis – stockings, minihep.
5. Urinary catheter if jaundiced.
6. Position supine on X-ray table with image intensifier available.

Procedure

Options for incision include the classical Kocher's, a mini-Kocher's, paramedian, midline or right upper transverse. The authors recommend the latter.

For a transverse incision, incise the skin and subcutaneous tissues, then divide the anterior rectus sheath in the line of the skin incision. Pass a large forceps behind the rectus to pull a swab through as this protects the deeper layers. Use diathermy to cut through the muscle. Take care to identify all vessels before they retract into the cut ends of the muscle.

Divide and ligate the falciform ligament and perform a laparotomy. Run a hand over the right lobe of the liver to introduce air as this helps the exposure. Use warm moist abdominal towels to pack the colon and stomach from the field of vision and carefully retract the liver to optimise exposure. Place a sponge-holding forceps on the fundus and a second on Hartmann's pouch. Hold the instruments in your non-dominant hand and carefully divide the peritoneum over the cystic duct.

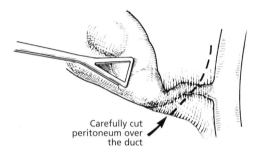

Carefully cut peritoneum over the duct

Fig. 5.25

Tease the adventitial tissue away from the cystic duct using a pledget and gently pass the tips of a forceps beneath it.

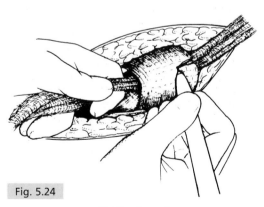

Fig. 5.24

Dividing the rectus

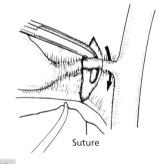

Suture

Fig. 5.26

Divide the posterior leaflet of peritoneum and carefully pass an absorbable suture behind the duct.

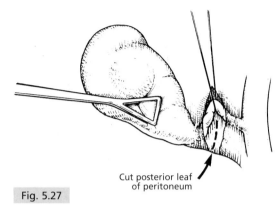

Fig. 5.27

Cut posterior leaf of peritoneum

The junction of the cystic duct with the common bile duct should now be visible. Once you are satisfied with the anatomical demonstration the cystic duct may be ligated. Place the proximal ligature as close as possible to the gallbladder and the second suture a few millimetres distal to this. If cholangiography is to be performed the distal suture should be placed but not tied.

Operative cholangiography

Introduce a cholangiogram catheter via a small incision in the cystic duct wall and once it is in position tie the ligature.

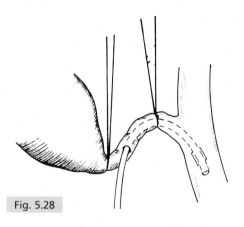

Fig. 5.28

If it is impossible to cannulate the cystic duct, tie the distal suture and carefully introduce a 25-gauge needle into the common bile duct.

Tilt the left side of the table upward by 10–15 degrees so as not to project the biliary tree over the spine. Screen the patient whilst 10 ml of radio-opaque dye is injected.

Identify, ligate and divide the cystic artery as it runs across Calot's triangle.

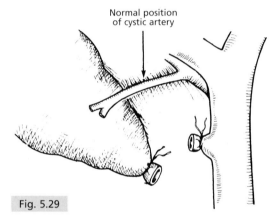

Normal position of cystic artery

Fig. 5.29

Dissect the gallbladder away from the liver using scissors or diathermy. Do not be tempted to use fingers for blunt dissection as this leaves a raw surface that will bleed. It is better to leave the serosa than to cut into the hepatic parenchyma.

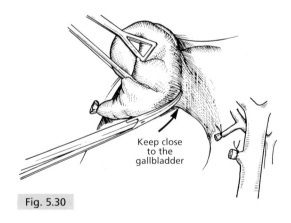

Keep close to the gallbladder

Fig. 5.30

Common bile duct exploration

If stones are identified they should be removed. Place fine stay sutures in the wall of the common bile duct and make a longitudinal incision between them just above the duodenum.

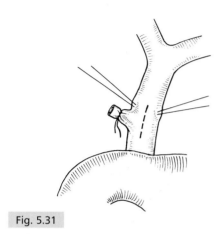

Fig. 5.31

Small stones may be flushed out with the aid of saline introduced through a fine catheter.

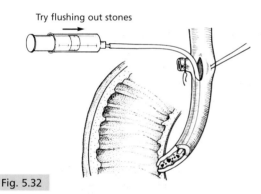

Try flushing out stones

Fig. 5.32

Larger stones may require a Fogarty catheter or a Desjardins's forceps. Check with a choledochoscope that all the stones have been extracted.

When the duct is clear and there is good flow of contrast to the duodenum introduce a T tube into the bile duct and exit it through the abdominal wall. Test the patency of the T tube by injecting a small volume of saline. Once complete, close the duct with fine interrupted absorbable sutures.

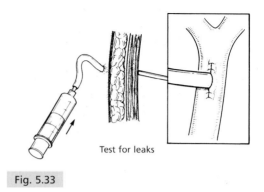

Test for leaks

Fig. 5.33

Bleeding can be arrested with controlled use of diathermy. If a small amount of oozing persists then a piece of Kaltostat may be placed on the liver bed. When haemostasis is satisfactory place a suction drain in the gallbladder fossa and close the wound.

Key points

1. The secret to exposing the junction of the cystic and common bile ducts is to place tension on the cystic duct. As the operation proceeds the view may be improved by repositioning of the forceps.
2. Do not cut or tie until you are entirely happy with the anatomy.
3. The introduction of the tips of a pair of artery forceps into the cystic duct will make it easier to cannulate.
4. If a cholangiogram is being performed be careful not to introduce air, as air bubbles may be difficult to distinguish from small calculi.
5. If you are unable to dislodge an impacted stone from the common duct seek assistance as a duodenotomy and sphincterotomy or choledoche-duodenostomy may be required. Alternatively this may be performed postoperatively via ERCP.
6. An alternative technique, which is particularly useful in the case of difficult anatomy, is a retrograde dissection of the gallbladder. This releases the gallbladder, allowing a thorough evaluation of the anatomy, leaving ligation of the vessels as the final step.

Indications

1. Elective   Haematological disorders.
   Part of radical upper abdominal surgery.
   Cysts/tumours of spleen.
   Staging of lymphoma (rarely performed).
2. Emergency Trauma.

The approach to the ruptured spleen differs from that of an elective splenectomy. Patients suffering splenic trauma should initially be managed as for the ATLS protocol with control of the airway, breathing and circulation (ABC). Peritoneal lavage or radiological imaging should be used to assess intra-abdominal injuries prior to surgery.

Setting up

1. General anaesthetic.
2. Nasogastric tube.
3. Antibiotic prophylaxis.
4. Anti-DVT prophylaxis – stockings, minihep.
5. Supine position.

Procedure

An upper left paramedian, midline, transverse or left subcostal incision may be utilised. In the case of trauma the midline incision allows improved access to the other viscera.

Elective splenectomy

The first and most important step is division of the lienorenal ligament. Standing on the right of the patient, and with the assistant carefully retracting the left margin of the wound, pass a hand over the spleen down to the lienorenal ligament. Gently retract the spleen and divide the lienorenal ligament, starting from the lower and moving towards the upper pole, using long-handled scissors.

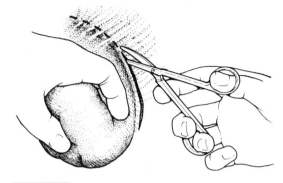

Fig. 5.34

Now pull up on the spleen with your non-dominant hand and gently push away the peritoneum with a swab on a stick. Continue sweeping away the tissues from behind the spleen as it is delivered up into the wound. The omentum can then be detached from the lower pole by division of the left gastroepiploic vessels between artery forceps and ligation with absorbable ties. At this stage the short gastric vessels passing from the upper pole of the spleen to the stomach through the gastrosplenic ligament should be individually ligated and divided. Care must be taken not to damage the stomach.

Attention is then turned to the main splenic vessels. Pass a couple of fingers of the non-dominant hand around the hilum and palpate the branches of the splenic artery as they pass into the spleen. With your thumb on the tail of the pancreas to protect it, clip and divide these branches together with their veins.

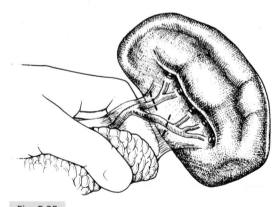

Fig. 5.35

Residual gastrosplenic ligament can then be divided. The spleen can now be removed and the main vessels double-ligated, the artery before the vein. A suction drain is placed in the subphrenic space and the abdominal wall closed in layers.

Emergency splenectomy

In the case of a ruptured spleen extensive haemorrhage may obscure the view obtained. The first procedure is to evacuate the clot both manually and with the aid of suction. Pass your hand down to the hilum to gain control of the haemorrhage by applying pressure to the splenic artery and vein between finger and thumb. If there is continued bleeding control may be achieved by applying a non-crushing intestinal clamp to the hilum. This allows time for assessment of the degree of splenic damage. If conservation is not possible then a formal splenectomy should be performed.

If at laparotomy bleeding is seen to originate from a single laceration then this may simply be sutured (splenorrhaphy). Alternatively, if there is a completely or partially avulsed fragment of spleen, a partial splenectomy may be performed by dividing the splenic vessels supplying the pole in question, resecting the fragment and oversewing the edge with absorbable mattress sutures. Decapsulating injuries such as ruptured subcapsular haematomas may be managed by application of topical haemostatic agents and wrapping the spleen in absorbable mesh.

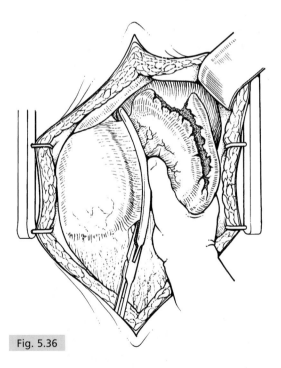

Fig. 5.36

Key points

1. Care is required in handling the spleen at all times.
2. Haemostasis is of vital importance no matter what is the indication for splenectomy.
3. Take care not to damage the pancreas during dissection of the splenic hilum.
4. Splenunculi are not uncommon and should be removed except in the case of trauma.
5. Vaccination against *Streptococcus pneumoniae* and *Haemophilus influenzae B* should be performed 6 weeks prior to operation for elective cases and as soon as possible postoperatively in the case of emergency splenectomy.
6. Splenectomised patients should also receive long-term prophylaxis against pneumococcal sepsis with phenoxymethyl penicillin (250 mg b.d.).
7. In view of the risk of postsplenectomy sepsis the splenic tissue should be preserved wherever possible in cases of trauma.
8. With large spleens the operation is facilitated by preliminary ligation of the splenic artery in continuity as it runs along the upper border of the pancreas. This rapidly 'deflates' the spleen.

6

LOWER GASTROINTESTINAL

APPENDICECTOMY

Indications

1. Emergency – acute appendicitis.
2. Elective – 'interval' appendicectomy after initial conservative treatment of an appendix mass.

Setting up

1. General anaesthetic.
2. Prophylactic antibiotics.
3. Supine position.

Procedure

The common incisions for appendicectomy are shown in Fig. 1.1. The classical incision is made at McBurney's point – an anatomical landmark two-thirds of the way along a straight line drawn between the umbilicus and the anterior superior iliac spine. The incision is made at 90° to this imaginary line.

The Lanz incision '4' is cosmetically superior, and by pulling the skin up towards the costal margin prior to incision will produce a scar lower down over the anterior abdominal wall. In the middle-aged or elderly patient a lower transverse or midline incision should be considered if the diagnosis is in doubt.

Incise the external oblique aponeurosis in the line of its fibres, exposing the internal oblique. If you are too medial you will see the rectus sheath. Split the

internal oblique fibres transversely with scissors and complete the split using fingers or a pair of retractors to enlarge the defect.

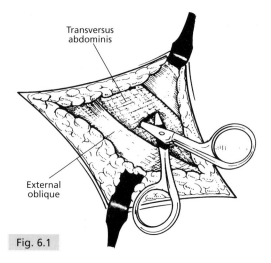

Fig. 6.1

Pick up the peritoneum between two fine clips and incise it with a scalpel. A gush of turbid fluid indicates appendicitis.

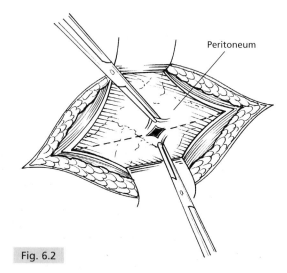

Fig. 6.2

The omentum may also be immediately present in acute appendicitis. Take a pus sample for culture and sensitivity.

Identify the caecum from its taeniae, and deliver it into the wound along with the appendix. If the appendix is retrocaecal or pelvic in position, 'winkle' it out using the index finger of your dominant hand. If it still is not possible to deliver the appendix into the wound enlarge the incision. This is best done by dividing fibres of the internal oblique laterally and medially. In obese patients the rectus sheath can also be incised to allow adequate exposure.

Having delivered the appendix, hold it with two tissue forceps. Divide the meso-appendix between artery clips, tying the pedicles with absorbable sutures.

Apply a purse-string or 'Z' stitch to the base of the appendix using a 2/0 absorbable suture. Crush the base of the appendix using a heavy forceps and ligate it proximally with a size 0 absorbable suture.

Remove the appendix and bury the stump by tightening the purse-string stitch. A useful tip is to hold the ligated base under the purse-string and push down as the purse-string is drawn tight.

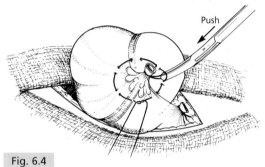

Push

Fig. 6.4

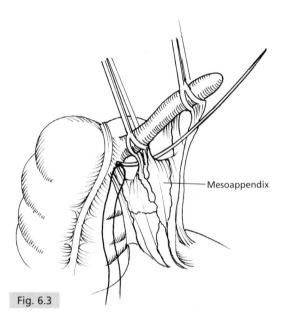

Mesoappendix

Fig. 6.3

Suck out any remaining free fluid and wash out the peritoneal cavity. Close the abdominal wall in layers using absorbable sutures. Use a continuous suture for the peritoneum and approximate the internal oblique with interrupted sutures. Repair the defect in the external oblique with a continuous suture and the skin with a subcuticular suture.

Key points

1. If there is an abscess present and the appendix cannot be found, place a drain to the abscess and close the abdomen.
2. If you find a carcinoma of the caecum seek assistance and perform a right hemicolectomy (see p. 71).
3. If the appendix is normal look for a Meckel's diverticulum, gynaecological pathology or sigmoid diverticulitis. If you find a gynaecological problem call for specialist help.
4. In a child carefully observe the ileal mesentery for enlarged lymph nodes – mesenteric adenitis.
5. In a true retrocaecal appendix the caecum can be mobilised by dividing its lateral peritoneal attachments as for a right hemicolectomy.

SMALL BOWEL RESECTION

Indications

1. Ischaemia, mesenteric infarction, necrosis following strangulation by a band or hernia.
2. Meckel's diverticulum.
3. Small bowel trauma.
4. Small bowel obstruction, e.g. secondary tumour or intussusception.

Setting up

1. General anaesthetic.
2. Nasogastric tube.
3. Prophylactic antibiotics.
4. Supine position.

Procedure

Through a midline incision deliver the diseased segment into the wound. Protect the wound edges with swabs to minimise sepsis. Use two non-crushing clamps to occlude the bowel either side of the diseased segment.

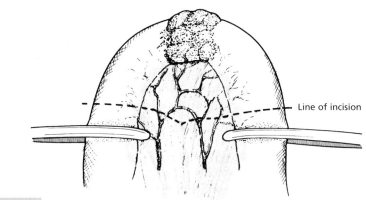

Line of incision

Fig. 6.5

Carefully incise the peritoneum of the mesentery along the line chosen for division of the vessels. Find the enclosed mesenteric vessels by transilluminating the mesentery and divide between artery forceps, ligating with absorbable sutures.

Place crushing clamps at a 30° angle to the bowel and divide close to the clamp. This allows better perfusion of the anti-mesenteric border. Cut across the bowel with a knife and, having removed the diseased section of bowel, cover the cut ends of the remaining bowel with antiseptic-soaked swabs.

Begin the posterior wall of the anastomosis by inserting a seromuscular continuous absorbable suture.

Following this, starting in the midline, insert a full-thickness double-ended absorbable suture. Sew towards the mesenteric margin and then 'around the corner' with one end of the suture. Then switch to the second layer and complete the anastomosis, tying the sutures in the midline anteriorly.

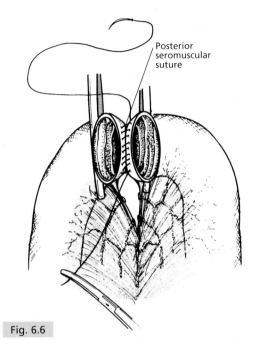

Posterior seromuscular suture

Fig. 6.6

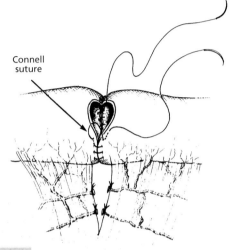

Connell suture

Fig. 6.7

Complete the anastomosis by inserting an anterior seromuscular suture.

Close the defect in the mesentery with interrupted absorbable sutures, taking care to avoid mesenteric vessels.

Close the abdominal wall as for laparotomy.

Key points

1. If the bowel ends do not bleed freely, resect them until healthy bowel is reached.
2. If the completed anastomosis looks dusky and does not improve after a few minutes' observation, excise it and do it again.
3. Do not place occlusive clamps across the mesentery.

Indications

1. Acute inflammation.
2. Haemorrhage.
3. Internal obstruction due to a band.
4. Intussusception.

Setting up

1. General anaesthetic.
2. Supine position.
3. Nasogastric tube.
4. Prophylactic antibiotics.

Procedure

Through a midline incision deliver the segment of bowel bearing the diverticulum into the wound and isolate it from the remainder of the bowel with gauze towels. The diverticulum often has a prominent blood supply which must be carefully identified, ligated and divided.

Apply two crushing clamps across the diverticulum and two non-crushing clamps across the bowel.

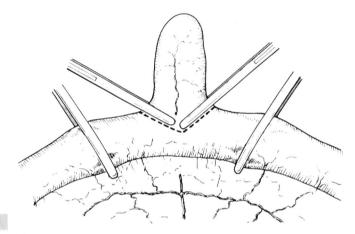

Fig. 6.8

Excise the diverticulum and close the resulting defect transversely using an interrupted 2/0 absorbable suture, and then insert a seromuscular layer on top.

Key points

1. A large diverticulum may require a formal small bowel resection, particularly if the base is thickened or abnormal.

Indications

1. Carcinoma of the caecum or of the ascending or transverse colon.
2. Crohn's disease, solitary diverticulum, intussusception.
3. Angiodysplasia of the colon.

Setting up

1. General anaesthetic.
2. Nasogastric tube.
3. Antibiotic prophylaxis.
4. Anti-DVT prophylaxis – stockings, minihep.
5. Urinary catheter.
6. Supine position.

Procedure

A midline incision is usual but a transverse muscle-cutting incision in the right iliac fossa can be less painful and is suitable in slimmer patients undergoing local resections.

Mobilise the caecum and terminal ileum by dividing the lateral peritoneum and continue mobilising clockwise up towards and including the gastrocolic omentum and the hepatic flexure.

Lift the right colon into the wound and sweep away any posterior tethering by blunt dissection with a 'swab on a stick'. Be careful to identify the gonadal vessels, the right ureter and the duodenum during this manoeuvre.

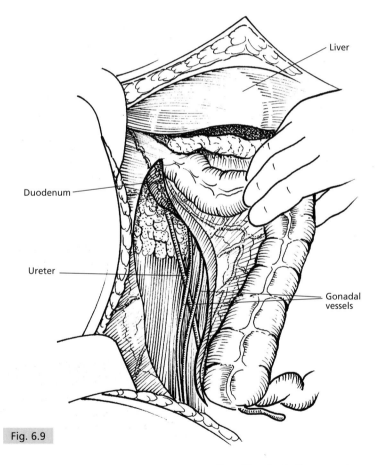

Liver

Duodenum

Ureter

Gonadal vessels

Fig. 6.9

Transilluminate the mesentery and ligate the vessels close to their origin with the superior mesenteric vessels if the operation is for tumour. Take the division of vessels up to the bowel wall.

LOWER GASTROINTESTINAL

Place non-crushing clamps on the transverse colon and ileum and divide the bowel between crushing clamps.

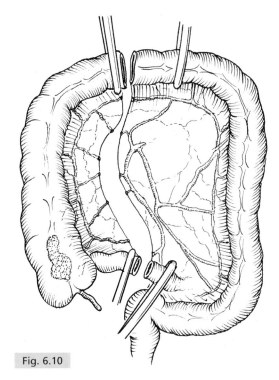

Fig. 6.10

Close the distal colon by hand or by using a mechanical stapling device and oversew the staple line. Approximate the ileum with the colon and commence the posterior wall by inserting a seromuscular suture.

Keep the sutures loose

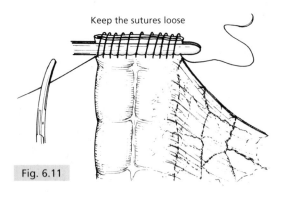

Fig. 6.11

Open the colon along its taeniae and insert a full-thickness absorbable suture to complete the posterior wall of the anastomosis using a double-ended suture commencing one way and then going the other way.

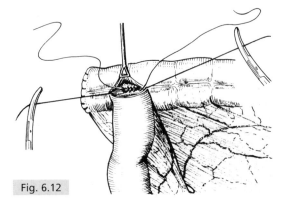

Fig. 6.12

Continue to the midline anterior and tie the sutures anteriorly and complete the anterior wall with a seromuscular suture.

Close the mesenteric defects and irrigate the peritoneal cavity. Close the wound in the conventional manner.

Key points

1. Do not anastomose bowel of doubtful viability.
2. Do not anastomose bowel under tension.
3. Confirm the presence of the ureter by gently pinching it between forceps and watching it 'wriggle'.
4. The procedure can be readily extended into distal colon as far as necessary should unexpected pathology be discovered at the time of laparotomy.
5. Alternative methods for anastomosis include end-to-end (useful if bowel diameters are comparable) and side-to-side (safest if bowel viability is in question). In addition the procedure can be accomplished entirely using stapling devices.
6. Beware of inadvertently ligating the superior mesenteric vessels.

Indications

1. Carcinoma.
2. Diverticular disease.
3. Colitis.

Setting up

1. General anaesthetic.
2. Nasogastric tube.
3. Antibiotic prophylaxis.
4. Anti-DVT prophylaxis – stockings, minihep.
5. Urinary catheter.
6. Supine position.
7. On-table irrigation if preoperative mechanical preparation is not possible.

Procedure

Enter the peritoneal cavity through a midline incision. Place the patient head-down and pack off the small bowel, using a self-retaining retractor.

Mobilise the colon by dividing along the 'white line of Toldt' with diathermy.

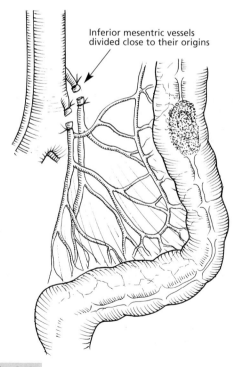

Inferior mesentric vessels divided close to their origins

Fig. 6.13

Push the sigmoid mesentery medially and identify the gonadal vessels and the left ureter as it crosses the pelvic brim. Use a swab on a stick to free-up any posterior attachments that may be present. Continue anti-clockwise up to the transverse colon.

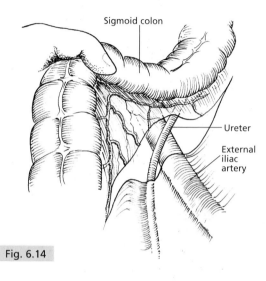

Sigmoid colon

Ureter

External iliac artery

Fig. 6.14

Transilluminate the mesentery and identify and ligate the vessels close to their origin. Distally, ligate the vessels at the bowel wall.

Place non-crushing clamps across the rectum and proximal bowel and crushing clamps at the points of resection. Protect the wound edges from contamination using abdominal swabs and place an antiseptic-soaked swab behind the intended points of transection. Using a knife, excise the disease segment of colon and cover the ends with the antiseptic swabs.

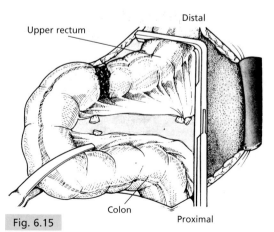

Upper rectum

Distal

Colon

Proximal

Fig. 6.15

Anastomosis is best accomplished by a single-layer technique. Insert a series of interrupted non-absorbable sutures in the posterior wall and when all are present tie them in sequence with the knots on the inside.

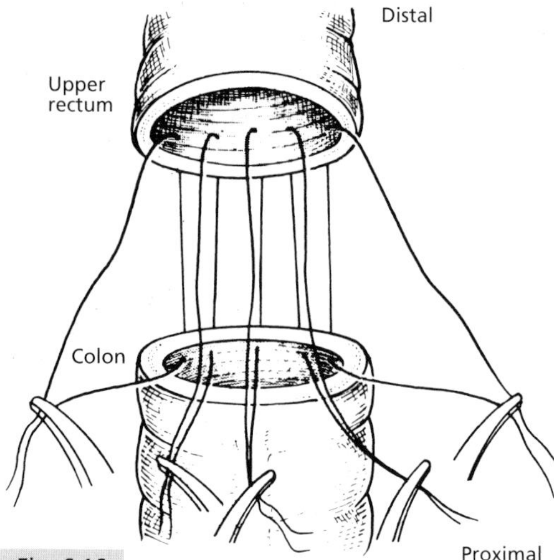

Close the mesenteric defect and wash out the peritoneal cavity. Insert a suction drain into the pelvis if there is sepsis present or there has been excessive oozing. Close the wound as for laparotomy.

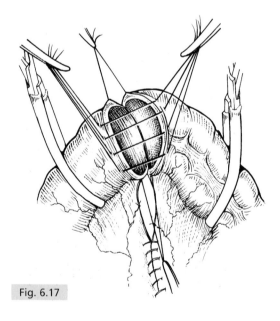

Distal

Upper
rectum

Colon

Proximal

Fig. 6.16

Full thickness technique

Complete the anterior wall in a similar fashion, this time knotting on the outside.

Key points

1. The anastomosis must be tension-free. Mobilise more proximal colon if there is a problem.
2. If the sigmoid tumour is adherent to the pelvic wall seek help, as complete excision of a tumour by removal of adjacent tissue determines the chance of cure.
3. A primary anastomosis should not be attempted in the presence of bowel obstruction or severe sepsis unless on-table irrigation has been performed. If you have no experience of this perform a Hartmann's procedure.
4. Do not pull down whilst mobilising the transverse colon or you may tear the spleen.
5. It is always wise to discuss the possibility of a stoma with the patient before operating, especially if there is any doubt regarding the precise nature of the colonic pathology.
6. An interrupted technique exluding the mucosa (serosubmucosal) can also be used. An alternative technique for anastomosis is a two-layer approach comprising full-thickness and seromuscular layers.

Fig. 6.17

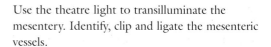

Indications

1. Obstructing lesion in the sigmoid colon.
2. Perforated lesion in the sigmoid colon.
3. Volvulus of the sigmoid colon.

Setting up

1. General anaesthetic.
2. Nasogastric tube.
3. Antibiotic prophylaxis.
4. Anti-DVT prophylaxis – stockings, minihep.
5. Urinary catheter.
6. Supine position.
7. On-table irrigation if pre-operative mechanical preparation is not possible.

Procedure

Through a midline incision mobilise the sigmoid colon as for a left hemicolectomy. Start by dividing the lateral peritoneum along its 'white line', which should be an avascular plane.

Sweep the sigmoid mesentery medially using a 'swab on a stick' and identify the gonadal vessels and the left ureter.

Use the theatre light to transilluminate the mesentery. Identify, clip and ligate the mesenteric vessels.

Place non-crushing clamps across the distal and proximal bowel and crushing clamps at the limits of the resection. Protect the wound edges from contamination using abdominal swabs and place an antiseptic-soaked swab behind the intended points of transection. Using a knife, excise the disease segment of colon and cover the ends with the antiseptic swabs.

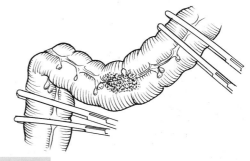

Fig. 6.19

Close the distal colon with two layers of continuous sutures. Alternatively, a linear cutting/stapling device can be used to both transect and close the distal bowel.

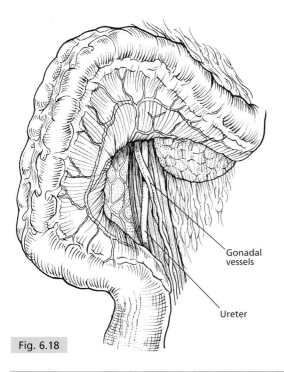

Gonadal vessels

Ureter

Fig. 6.18

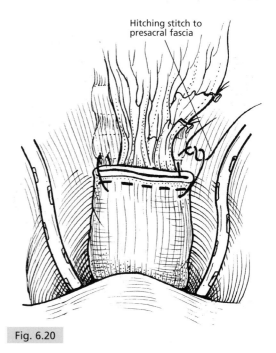

Hitching stitch to presacral fascia

Fig. 6.20

Bring out the colon proximal to the lesion as an end stoma. Make a circular incision in the skin, approximately 2 cm in diameter, and deepen it down to the rectus sheath. Palpate the inferior epigastric vessels to avoid damage at this stage.

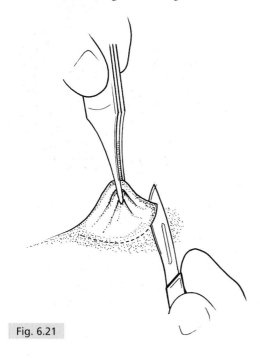

Fig. 6.21

Make a cruciate incision in the sheath and bluntly dissect through the muscle into the peritoneal cavity.

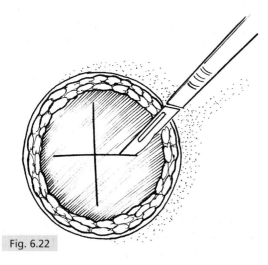

Fig. 6.22

Place a clamp through the stoma site and capture the proximal colon. Gently manipulate the bowel through the abdominal wall.

Wash out the peritoneal cavity, insert a suction drain in the pelvis and close the abdominal wall prior to completing the stoma. Place clean towels around the wound site.

Approximate the skin and bowel wall edge with interrupted absorbable sutures. Place sutures around the circumference at regular intervals.

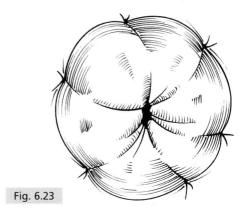

Fig. 6.23

When finished, clean the wound thoroughly and apply a colostomy bag.

Key points

1. If the rectal stump is long and re-anastomosis is anticipated, tack up to the abdominal wall to aid fixing it at the second operation.
2. Always try to optimise the stoma position preoperatively with the assistance of a stomatherapist.
3. Take care not to twist the bowel or place undue tension on the bowel when constructing the stoma as this will compromise its vascularity.
4. A sigmoid volvulus often continues as a megarectum, making closure of the rectal stump difficult.
5. This operation has a very high wound-infection rate. Repeated lavage with tetracycline (1 g/litre) throughout the procedure combined with intravenous antibiotics minimises the complication.
6. It is well worth hitching the distal bowel to the presacral fascia so as to make identification of the bowel easier in the case of reversal of the Hartmann's procedure.

Indications

A permanent colostomy following abdominoperineal resection of the rectum.

Setting up

1. General anaesthetic.
2. Nasogastric tube.
3. Antibiotic prophylaxis.
4. Anti-DVT prophylaxis – stockings, minihep.
5. Urinary catheter.
6. Supine position.

Procedure

An end colostomy is always formed as part of a major abdominal procedure. Construction of the stoma is not commenced until the primary procedure has been completed. End colostomies are usually formed in the left lower quadrant. Before making the skin incision place some forceps on the edge of the abdominal wound and pull towards the midline – this helps correct placement of the skin wound.

Pick up the skin and excise a 2 cm disc; excise a cylinder of tissue down to the rectus sheath (Fig. 6.21). Divide the sheath in a cruciate manner and with blunt dissection through the muscle as far as the peritoneum (Fig. 6.22).

Enlarge the defect as necessary with manual traction using your fingers. Palpate the inferior epigastric vessels to avoid damage or haematoma.

It is good practice for permanent colostomies to pass the colon through the peritoneum at a point lateral to the intended stoma site as this creates a tunnel which should reduce the incidence of stomal herniation.

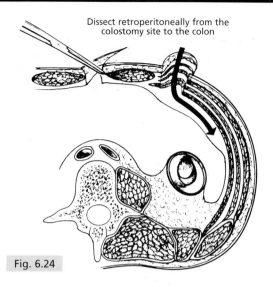

Dissect retroperitoneally from the colostomy site to the colon

Fig. 6.24

Feed the colon through the incision, taking care not to twist it. Insert six to eight sutures between the external oblique aponeurosis and the colon to prevent stomal retraction or prolapse. Approximate the skin and bowel wall edge with interrupted absorbable sutures placed at 3, 6, 9 and 12 o'clock positions. Insert further sutures at regular intervals.

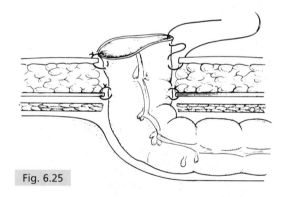

Fig. 6.25

When finished, clean the wound thoroughly and apply a colostomy bag.

Key points

1. Necrosis and retraction can be avoided by absence of tension, and a good blood supply to the end of the colon.
2. Proper siting by a stomatherapist is mandatory in elective cases. Remember not to wash off this mark when preparing the abdomen prior to incision.
3. Close the abdomen and cover the wound before opening and suturing the colostomy.

FORMATION OF A LOOP COLOSTOMY

Indications

1. To defunction an obstructed colon.
2. As a temporary bypass after a more distal bowel anastomosis.

Setting up

1. General anaesthetic.
2. Nasogastric tube.
3. Antibiotic prophylaxis.
4. Anti-DVT prophylaxis – stockings, minihep.
5. Urinary catheter.
6. Supine position.

Procedure

It is unusual to have to perform a 'blind' loop colostomy without a concomitant laparotomy. However, both the above can be performed through small incisions in each area.

There are two main sites for loop colostomies. The first is in the right transverse colon through the right upper abdominal area. The second is in the sigmoid colon in the left iliac fossa.

Pick up the preoperatively marked skin and excise a 2 cm disc continuing down to the rectus sheath (Fig. 6.21).

Make a cruciate incision in the sheath and dissect the muscle bluntly down to the peritoneum (Fig. 6.22). Use two-finger traction to enlarge the defect as required.

For a transverse colostomy, dissect some of the greater omentum away from the transverse colon and open up a window in the mesentery. Pass a length of soft rubber tubing, e.g. a Foley catheter, through the window. By applying gentle traction to

Key points

1. It is most important to have the stoma site properly marked preoperatively by the stomatherapist whenever possible.
2. Do not site the stoma in the left upper quadrant if at all possible as the left transverse colon/splenic flexure is the site of watershed of the arterial supply.
3. Remove the colostomy bridge after 7–10 days.

the rubber sling deliver the colon through the abdominal wall.

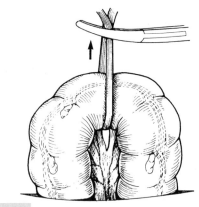

Fig. 6.26

When the colon is in position, exchange the rubber for a colostomy bridge.

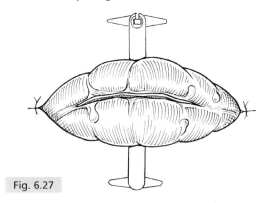

Fig. 6.27

Open the bowel longitudinally along the taenia with a knife to allow any explosive gases to be released, and then open the incision with diathermy. Suture the edges of the stoma to the skin edges using regularly placed interrupted absorbable sutures.

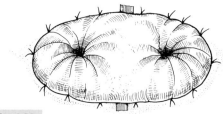

Fig. 6.28

Clean the skin and fit an appropriate colostomy appliance.

Indications

1. To restore bowel continuity after temporary faecal diversion.
2. Prior to operation it is important to examine radiologically the integrity of the distal anastomosis to ensure no leakage or stenosis.

Setting up

1. General anaesthetic.
2. Nasogastric tube.
3. Antibiotic prophylaxis.
4. Anti-DVT prophylaxis – stockings, minihep.
5. Urinary catheter.
6. Supine position.

Procedure

Incise around the stoma about 0.5 cm from the mucocutaneous edge. Place forceps on this edge and apply traction upwards.

Deepen the incision and angle inwards towards the colon, taking care not to breach the bowel wall.

Continue this process until the colon is free all the way around.

Excise the old stoma and close the colon with interrupted 2/0 full-thickness absorbable sutures.

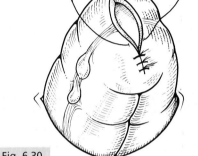

Fig. 6.30

Close the abdominal-wall muscle layer with interrupted non-absorbable sutures and interrupted sutures for the skin.

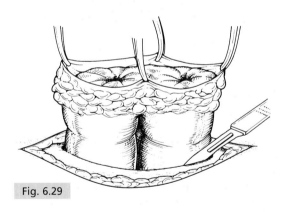

Fig. 6.29

Key points

1. Adequate mobilisation is vital; if necessary extend the skin incision to free-up more colon.
2. Closure of end colostomies is uncommon unless they are formed as part of a Hartmann's procedure; in this case the reversal of Hartmann's is a consultant procedure.
3. It is essential that the tissue of the colonic wall used for closure is soft and supple to avoid leakage. Excise all rugged and oedematous tissue.

Indications

As a permanent stoma after total colectomy.

Setting up

1. General anaesthetic.
2. Nasogastric tube.
3. Antibiotic prophylaxis.
4. Anti-DVT prophylaxis – stockings, minihep.
5. Urinary catheter.
6. Supine position.

Procedure

An end ileostomy is always constructed at the same time as a panproctocolectomy and is usually formed in the right iliac fossa.

Having excised the colon, ensure the ileum is cleared of its mesentery for several centimetres and that the ileum itself is viable.

Incise a 2 cm circle of skin at the appropriate location, over the outer half of the rectus, and continue the incision down to the rectus sheath (Fig. 6.21). Avoid the inferior epigastric vessels.

Make a cruciate incision in the sheath and use blunt dissection to split the muscle fibres down to the peritoneum (Fig. 6.22).

Place a tissue forceps through the stoma opening and grasp the ileum. Whilst taking care not to twist the bowel, gently manipulate it through the abdominal wall.

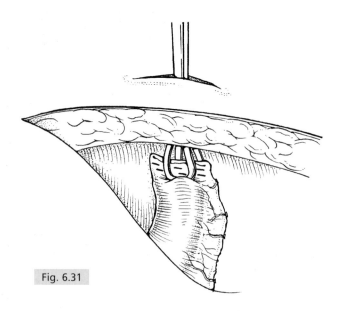

Fig. 6.31

Stitch the ileal serosa and mesentery to the anterior abdominal wall to close the mesenteric defect and prevent internal herniation.

Wash out the peritoneal cavity, insert a suction drain and close the abdominal wall. Place clean towels around the wound site.

It is important to make sure that you have 6–8 cm of ileum protruding beyond the skin surface so as to allow a spout to be created.

Insert eight equally spaced anchoring sutures between the ileum and the external oblique aponeurosis to prevent subsequent stomal prolapse; then approximate the skin and bowel wall edge with interrupted absorbable sutures.

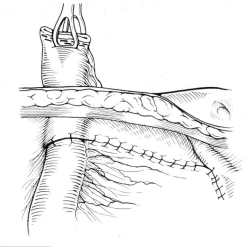

Fig. 6.32

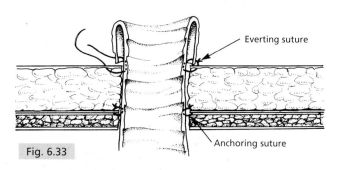

Everting suture

Anchoring suture

Fig. 6.33

When finished, apply an ileostomy appliance.

Key points

1. The ideal length of the spout should be 2–3 cm. If the everted ileum is significantly longer than this, trim a little of the ileum and reform the spout.
2. Complications of stomal construction including herniation, prolapse and retraction are largely due to poor surgical technique and can therefore be minimised (but not avoided) by paying attention to details.
3. The terminal ileum serves a very important absorptive function, so as little as possible should be excised.

Indications

Loop ileostomy is preferred to loop colostomy to defunction distal colorectal anastomoses.

Setting up

1. General anaesthetic.
2. Nasogastric tube.
3. Antibiotic prophylaxis.
4. Anti-DVT prophylaxis – stockings, minihep.
5. Urinary catheter.
6. Supine position.

Procedure

A loop ileostomy is constructed following a colonic resection and distal colorectal or colo-anal anastomosis and therefore a laparotomy will already have been performed.

Make a transverse incision over the preoperatively determined site, usually the right lower quadrant. Incise a 2 cm circle of skin at the appropriate location and continue the incision down to the rectus sheath (Fig. 6.21).

Make a cruciate incision in the sheath and use blunt dissection to split the muscle fibres down to the peritoneum (Fig. 6.22).

Select an appropriate loop of ileum that will reach the stoma site without tension and mark the

proximal limb of the loop with a stitch. Open a window in its mesentery and pass a length of rubber tubing through the defect.

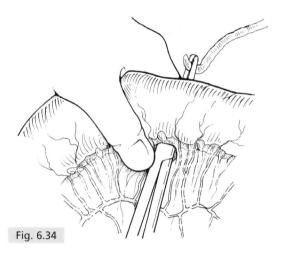

Fig. 6.34

Place a tissue forceps through the stoma opening and grasp the ileum. Gently manipulate it through the abdominal wall whilst taking care not to twist the bowel. When this is done, replace the rubber tube with an ileostomy bridge.

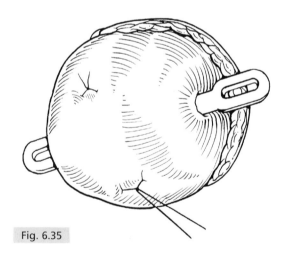

Fig. 6.35

Complete the primary procedure by washing out the peritoneal cavity, inserting a suction drain and closing the abdominal wall. Place clean towels around the wound site.

Open the ileum by incising the bowel for half its circumference, using diathermy at a point 2 cm from the level of the skin in the distal limb.

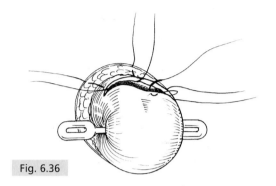

Fig. 6.36

Create a spout of ileum on the proximal section of the loop by inserting a pair of tissue forceps into the lumen and gently grasping the mucosa. Using dissecting forceps carefully peel back the bowel until the ileal spout has been created.

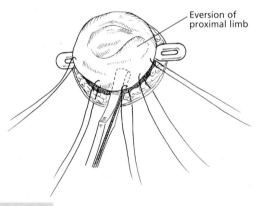

Eversion of proximal limb

Fig. 6.37

Insert three or four interrupted absorbable sutures to secure the defunctioned side of the stoma to the skin and six to eight on the functioning side.

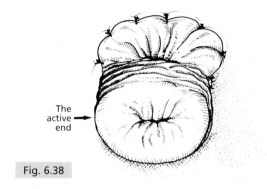

The active end →

Fig. 6.38

Apply an ileostomy appliance.

Key points

1. Take care to evert the proximal functioning loop, not the distal non-functioning loop.
2. Do not rotate more than 90° when drawing through the abdominal wall.
3. Try to evert 2–3 cm of ileum to aid the stomatherapist.

CLOSURE OF A LOOP ILEOSTOMY

Indications

To restore bowel continuity after temporary faecal diversion.

Setting up

1. General anaesthetic.
2. Nasogastric tube.
3. Antibiotic prophylaxis.
4. Anti-DVT prophylaxis – stockings, minihep.
5. Urinary catheter.
6. Supine position.

Procedure

Mobilisation of the stoma begins in a similar fashion to colostomy closure. Incise around the stoma about 0.5 cm from the mucocutaneous edge.

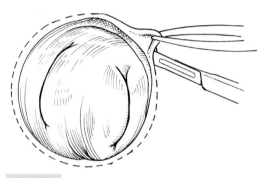

Fig. 6.39

Deepen the incision so as to free-up the two limbs of terminal ileum with their mucocutaneous junction.

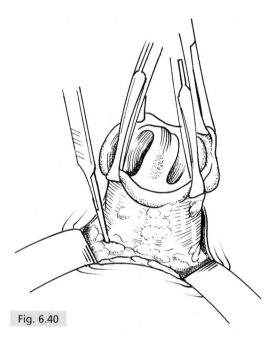

Fig. 6.40

It is important not to narrow the already small-calibre ileum when re-anastomosing the limbs. A stapling technique is therefore preferred to produce a side-to-side anastomosis. Using a linear stapler, and taking care not to include the mesentery in the staple line, staple the two limbs.

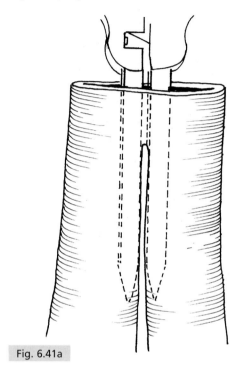

Fig. 6.41a

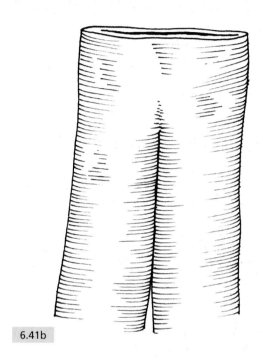

6.41b

Close and excise the old mucocutaneous junction by firing a cutting/stapling device across the open ends of the ileum.

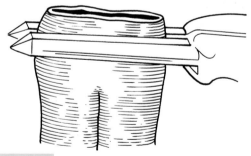

Fig. 6.42

Key points

1. Always check the integrity of the anastomosis prior to contemplating ileostomy closure.
2. Take care not to narrow the lumen or damage the mesenteric vessels when firing the stapling device.

Close the abdominal wall with interrupted non-absorbable sutures, and the skin with interrupted or continuous subcuticular absorbable sutures.

7

ANAL / PERIANAL

PROCTOSCOPY AND SIGMOIDOSCOPY

Indications

An adequate proctoscopy and sigmoidoscopy is mandatory before performing any perianal procedure. This can either be done in the outpatient setting or in the operating theatre if the patient is proceeding to a further operation.

Setting up

1. Left lateral position.

Procedure

Both proctoscopes and sigmoidoscopes come in metal (re-usable) and plastic (disposable) varieties and are introduced with their associated obturators.

The proctoscope carries a light and is useful for inspecting the anal canal and in diagnosing haemorrhoids. Both banding and injection of haemorrhoids can be achieved through the proctoscope.

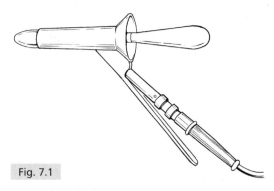

Fig. 7.1

The longer sigmoidoscope is used to examine the more proximal rectum, but rarely is one able to advance it further than this in the outpatient setting. It has an attached rubber air-pump bulb that allows inflation of the walls of the rectum. Biopsies can be achieved by detaching the window at the end of the sigmoidoscope and inserting long forceps under direct vision.

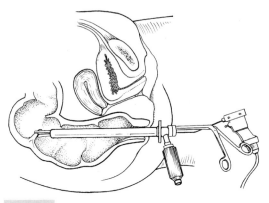

Fig. 7.2

Always perform a gentle rectal examination first, both for diagnostic purposes and to assess anal tenderness.

Then place the instrument against the sphincter and wait until it relaxes before introduction. Never force the instrument or cause excessive pain.

Key points

1. Always check the connections and light source before contemplating a procedure.
2. Do not attempt an examination in the outpatient department if you suspect an anal fissure. Instead perform the examination when the patient is under general anaesthetic.
3. Do not over-inflate the rectum, as this causes severe pain to the patient. It may also have disastrous consequences for your clothing when the scope is removed!
4. Examination with a flexible sigmoidoscope is preferable if an instrument is available, as it allows a more proximal visualisation of the colon.
5. Patients should ideally be given a microlax/phosphate enema when they first arrive in clinic, so as to ensure an adequate inspection of the mucosa.

Indications

Banding of haemorrhoids is employed in first- or second-degree haemorrhoids.

Setting up

1. Left lateral position.

Procedure

Having performed a full sigmoidoscopic examination, place a proctoscope in the anal canal. Gently withdraw the proctoscope until the pile groups are seen.

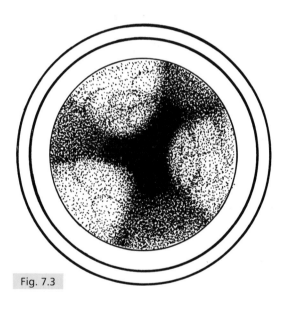

Fig. 7.3

Banding can be achieved by the suction bander or by the Baron's bander. The latter does not require an assistant to hold the proctoscope.

Grasp the pile group through the middle of the banding instrument and apply a band to the base of the pile.

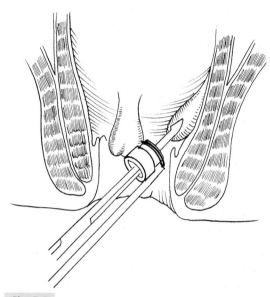

Fig. 7.4

A similar procedure can be done with the suction bander.

Two or three pile groups can be banded during a single outpatient visit.

Key points

1. It is important to counsel the patient beforehand and explain that this procedure can be painful afterwards.
2. Do not place bands too close to the dentate line as you may accidentally incorporate sensitive mucosa and cause severe pain.
3. Urinary retention can occur, and if the band is placed too superficially severe pain can ensue which requires removal of the band.
4. Bands are usually passed spontaneously a week or so later.
5. Laxatives should be employed to prevent constipation.

7 INJECTION OF HAEMORRHOIDS

Indications

1. First- or small second-degree piles.
2. Small mucosal prolapses.

Setting up

1. Left lateral position.

Procedure

With the patient in position, place the proctoscope in the anal canal.

Visualise the pile groups to be treated and inject 5% phenol in almond oil into their bases until the superficial tissues blanch, as this is an indication that the injection is in the correct plane.

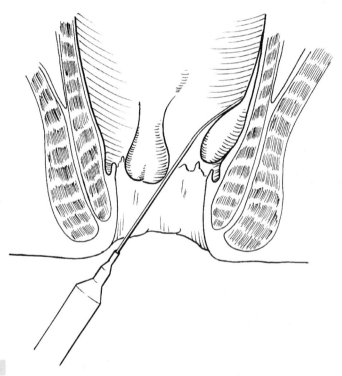

Fig. 7.5

Some 3 ml can be injected into each site.

Key points

1. Warn the patient beforehand that the procedure may be painful and that they may notice significant blood loss following the procedure.
2. Do not inject too close to the dentate line as you may cause severe pain.
3. Start with the lowest pile so that any bleeding does not obstruct the view.
4. Review in 6 weeks and reinject any haemorrhoids that remain.

Indications

Prolapsing (third-degree) piles.

Setting up

1. General anaesthetic.
2. Lithotomy position.

Procedure

Prior to performing a haemorrhoidectomy, thoroughly examine the patient and visualise the anal canal and rectum with a proctoscope. Confirm the position of the pile groups by introducing a dry gauze swab into the anal canal and gently withdrawing it.

Apply curved forceps to the perianal skin just outside the mucocutaneous junction at 3, 7 and 11 o'clock, opposite the primary pile groups. Retract on these forceps to bring the haemorrhoidal masses into view and apply a forceps to each. Commencing with the 7 o'clock group, insert an index finger into the rectum whilst holding the clips in the palm of the hand. Begin dissection with a U-shaped incision in the skin close to the pile.

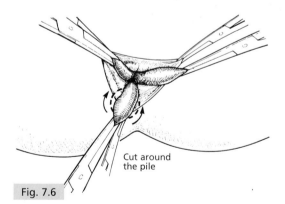

Cut around the pile

Fig. 7.6

Using a combination of blunt and sharp dissection, push the subcutaneous tissues towards the anal canal until the fibres of the internal sphincter are seen. Transfix and ligate the pile with an absorbable suture, leaving the suture ends long to aid identification in the case of bleeding.

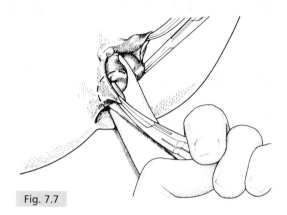

Fig. 7.7

Small bleeding points and tags can be dealt with now using diathermy. Repeat the same procedure for the remaining pile groups, leaving distinct skin bridges.

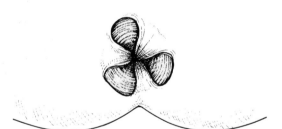

Fig. 7.8

'If it looks like a clover, the trouble is over'

At the end of the procedure place a soft petroleum jelly gauze or seaweed dressing in the anal canal. The patient will pass the swab after 24 hours.

Key points

1. Always do a sigmoidoscopy before the procedure even if somebody else has done it before.
2. Make sure that you are not too radical with the excisions; leave mucocutaneous bridges to prevent stenosis. If it looks like a clover the trouble is over, if it looks like a dahlia it's sure to be a failure!
3. Give postoperative stool softeners.
4. Bleeding must be completely controlled before leaving theatre, as haemorrhage from missed bleeding points can be profuse.

7 LATERAL INTERNAL SPHINCTEROTOMY

Indications

Chronic anal fissure.

Setting up

1. General anaesthetic.
2. Lithotomy position.

Procedure

First, perform a standard examination including proctoscopy and sigmoidoscopy to confirm the diagnosis as this will probably not have been possible in the outpatient department due to pain.

Introduce a bivalve anal retractor and palpate the lower edge of the internal sphincter at the 3 o'clock position.

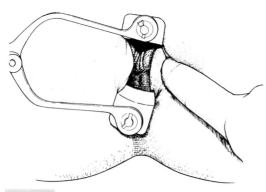

Fig. 7.9

Using a narrow-blade scalpel, incise the skin, keeping the blade between the skin and the internal sphincter. Rotate the scalpel to bring the cutting edge towards the sphincter and incise to the dentate line. Any residual fibres can be disrupted by finger pressure.

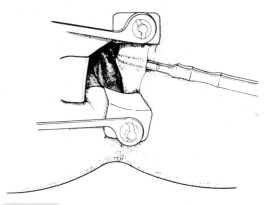

Fig. 7.10

Sphincterectomy with a knife

Infiltrate the incision with bupivicaine 0.25%.

Key points

1. Some fissures respond to non-operative conservative management with glyceryl trinitrate cream and stool softeners.
2. Postoperative stool softeners are necessary.
3. Warn the patient before the operation about the risks of transient incontinence for flatus particularly.
4. Anal stretching is no longer recommended.

Indications

1. Fistulae with persistent discharge.
2. Recurrent abscess formation in association with a fistula.

Setting up

1. General anaesthetic.
2. Lithotomy position or prone jack-knife position.

Procedure

Perform a full examination and sigmoidoscopy to inspect for internal openings of the fistula. Pass a probe very gently into the external fistulous opening and note the direction and depth in which the probe goes. Remember Goodsall's law when assessing the direction of the tract.

Provided the probe passes superficially the tract can now be excised. If the tract is deep the fistula is complex and specialist help is required.

To excise the fistula cut down on the probe and if necessary divide the superficial fibres of the internal sphincter.

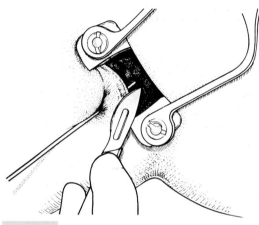

Fig. 7.12

Trim off any overhanging skin on either side of the fistula to encourage healing by granulation.

Apply an alginate dressing to aid haemostasis.

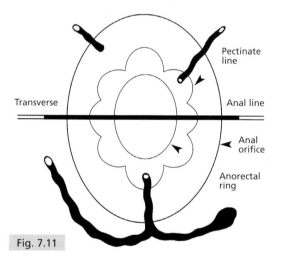

Pectinate line

Transverse

Anal line

Anal orifice

Anorectal ring

Fig. 7.11

Key points

1. If the patient has recurrent fistulae think of Crohn's disease and do not excise too much tissue.
2. Always send the excised tissue for histology.
3. If no help is available to deal with a high fistula, insert a nylon seton to aid drainage and reassess.
4. If the fistula is anything more than a simple low fistula seek expert assistance.

EVACUATION OF PERIANAL HAEMATOMA

Indications

Symptomatic haematoma.

Setting up

1. Local anaesthetic is preferred but a general anaesthetic may be required for nervous patients.
2. Left lateral position.

Procedure

Inject 5 ml of 1% lignocaine with adrenaline into the skin around the haematoma.

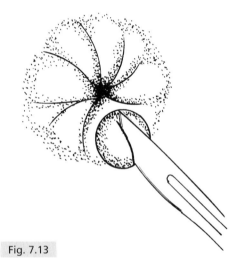

Fig. 7.13

Make a 1 cm incision on the surface of the haemorrhoid and evacuate the clot.

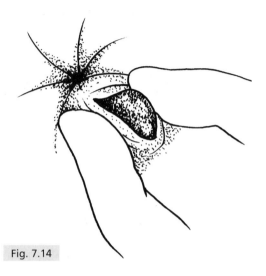

Fig. 7.14

Excise any redundant skin to reduce the risks of skin tag formation; then leave the wound to heal by secondary intention.

Key points

1. Prescribe a bulking agent to prevent constipation during the process of healing.

Indications

A perianal abscess that is 'pointing'. Ischio-rectal abscesses point further away from the anal margin and are dealt with similarly.

Setting up

1. General anaesthetic.
2. Lithotomy position.

Procedure

Perform a proctoscopic examination to inspect for internal fistulous openings. Incise the abscess and make a cruciate incision of about 2 cm.

Excise the resultant four skin edges and digitally break down any loculi of the abscess. Send pus and skin for culture and histology respectively.

Pack the wound with an alginate dressing.

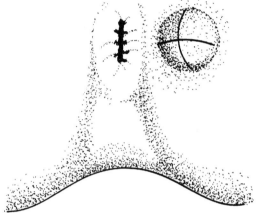

Fig. 7.15

Key points

1. If you find a fistula do not attempt to excise it at this first operation, as the anatomy can be difficult to assess in the presence of sepsis.
2. If you find pus coming from high up above the levator ani ask for specialist help.
3. If no fistula is evident, but the laboratory cultures coliforms from the abscess, a fistula is likely to be present, so consider anorectal ultrasound to look for a tract.

EXCISION OF PILONIDAL SINUS

Indications

A persistent or recurrent pilonidal sinus.

Setting up

1. General anaesthetic.
2. Prone jack-knife (or left lateral position) with buttock strapped apart.

Procedure

Pass a probe into the sinus and assess the number and direction of the tracts. Make an elliptical excision, incorporating all the openings.

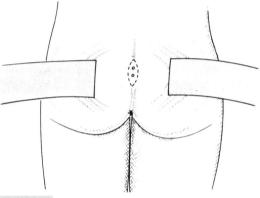

Fig. 7.16

Deepen the incision down to the sacral fascia and excise the block of tissue.

Use diathermy to achieve haemostasis. Excise any remote tracts via a separate incision.

Only small non-purulent sinuses should be closed in layers primarily. All others should be packed with seaweed dressing.

After some 48 hours this dressing can be changed for a silastic foam dressing which the patient can manage him- or herself.

Key points

1. Encourage the patient to keep the area hair-free by shaving.
2. Protracted healing can be due to low-grade sepsis. In this case, swab and treat with antibiotics.
3. An alternative procedure is to excise the sinuses and close the defect primarily.
4. Rotation flaps can also be used.

8
VASCULAR

Indications

1. Symptomatic varicose veins, with sapheno-femoral or sapheno-popliteal incompetence.
2. Cosmesis.
3. To assist varicose ulcer healing.

Setting up

1. General anaesthetic.
2. Supine position for long saphenous and prone for short saphenous veins with Trendelenburg position for high tie.
3. Prepare the legs from the abdomen to the heel.

Procedure

Long saphenous – Trendelenburg procedure

Make an incision in the skin crease 1.5 cm lateral and below the pubic tubercle.

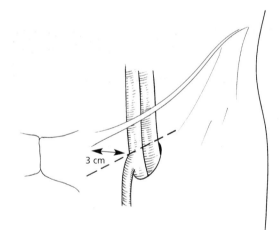

Fig. 8.1

Trace the long saphenous vein and its tributaries up to the sapheno-femoral junction.

Identify, ligate and divide all tributaries. The superficial external pudendal artery is invariably present; it can be divided if necessary.

Having ligated all the small tributaries, ligate the main sapheno-femoral junction, double-tying the vein proximally.

Long saphenous vein ready for ligation

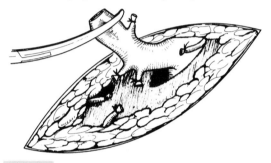

Fig. 8.2

Pass the vein stripper down the long saphenous vein to the knee and make a further skin incision to isolate the stripper. Identify the end of the stripper and, by applying gentle traction, strip the vein back up to the groin.

Close the small incision with steristrips. Use absorbable sutures to approximate the fascia of the groin incision with subcuticular sutures to the skin.

Avulse local varicosities in the lower calf through stab incisions using a small artery clip or vein hook to retrieve the vein. No ligations are usually necessary.

Short saphenous

It is not necessary to strip the short system. Use a preoperative Doppler scan to mark the sapheno-popliteal junction. Through a transverse skin incision trace the short saphenous vein to the popliteal junction and ligate the vein at the junction. Beware of the sural nerve lying lateral to the sapheno-popliteal junction.

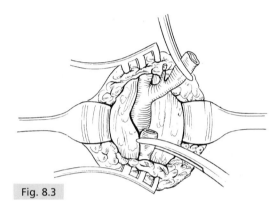

Fig. 8.3

Key points

1. Identify veins preoperatively with an indelible marker.
2. Take extreme care whilst dissecting the proximal long saphenous vein – do not blindly dissect around the sapheno femoral junction.
3. Encourage patients to mobilise as soon as is possible.
4. Recurrent veins should always be mapped with Doppler ultrasound.
5. Recurrent veins are a job for the boss!

Indications

Acute ischaemia of the lower limb.

Setting up

1. General anaesthetic.
2. Prone position.

Procedure

Feel for the femoral artery at the mid-inguinal point and make a longitudinal incision over it, extending the incision upwards across the skin crease of the groin.

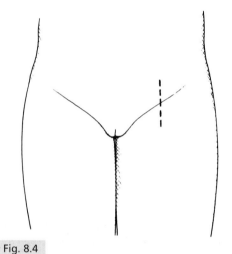

Fig. 8.4

Deepen the incision down to the inguinal ligament and then inset a self-retaining retractor. Identify the femoral artery just below the inguinal ligament, dissect it away from the surrounding fascia and pass a nylon tape or silicon sling around it.

Pull up on the sling and tease the tissues away from the artery using a small pledget held in artery forceps. Identify the superficial femoral artery, and then find the deep femoral (profunda) artery, which arises lateral and some 5 cm distal to the inguinal ligament. Pass a sling around each.

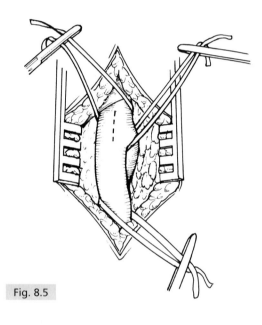

Fig. 8.5

The smaller arteries may be controlled by passing a ligature twice around each vessel and applying traction. Do not tie the ligatures but place a clip on each. Alternatively, small bulldog clips may be applied.

Place an angled vascular clamp (DeBakey) on each of the three main vessels and then make a longitudinal arteriotomy in the common femoral artery. Having tested the catheter balloon by injecting air or saline, deflate the balloon and pass the catheter proximally up to the aortic bifurcation as your assistant controls haemorrhage by tightening the uppermost tape. Inflate the balloon with one hand and remove the catheter with the other. Use just enough pressure to give some resistance as the balloon is withdrawn. Have your assistant relax on the tape to allow the balloon to emerge with any clot.

When you have good inflow, inject heparinised saline up the vessel and reapply the clamp. Repeat the procedure using a size 4 Fogarty catheter on the superficial and deep femoral arteries.

Having cleared all the vessels, repair the arteriotomy using a 5/0 non-absorbable suture. Remove the clamps and tapes, checking for haemostasis. Insert a suction drain alongside the catheter and close the wound with interrupted non-absorbable sutures.

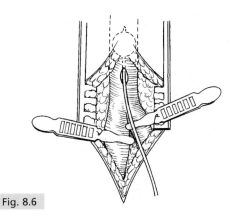

Fig. 8.6

Key points

1. The procedure may be performed under local anaesthetic in frail patients using 0.25% bupivicaine together with midazolam to provide sedation. However, an anaesthetist should always be present, as a general anaesthetic is preferable.
2. If there is underlying atheroma, a smaller Fogarty catheter may be required to clear the distal vessels.
3. If you cannot achieve good back-bleeding from the superficial and deep femoral arteries, perform an on-table angiogram.
4. If you cannot achieve good proximal flow call for assistance.
5. Do not over-distend the balloons as this may further damage the intima and lead to further thrombosis.
6. If you manage to retrieve an embolus as opposed to a simple blood clot send it for histological examination.
7. At the end of the procedure look for a clinical improvement in perfusion of the distal limb by checking and documenting the pulses.

1. Ischaemia or gangrene.
2. Trauma.
3. Tumours of bone or soft tissue.

The site of amputation has to be chosen carefully and may lie between the forefoot and the hip joint. Remember: the first amputation should be the last.

The two commonest procedures are above-knee and below-knee amputation.

Setting up

1. General anaesthetic.
2. Prone position.

Procedure

Above-knee amputation

The best place to divide the femur is 8–10 cm (one hand's breadth) above the upper border of the patella. Use a skin marker to plan your incisions, which should either make the anterior and posterior flaps of equal length or the anterior one slightly longer.

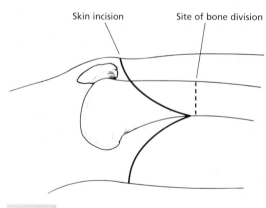

Fig. 8.7

Divide the skin and subcutaneous tissues along the planned lines. Achieving haemostasis is not usually a problem in ischaemic limbs but there may be profuse bleeding in septic limbs. Ligate all the veins using a 2/0 absorbable suture. Deepen the anterior incision down to bone, dividing the quadriceps tendon. Posteriorly, divide the muscles in a similar fashion. The femoral vessels, together with the medial and lateral popliteal nerves are found in a posteromedial position. Doubly ligate the vessels with an absorbable suture. Prior to dividing the nerves, apply tension to the nerves so that they retract into the stump upon division. If the amputation is performed at a higher level the sciatic nerve may be encountered. This has an accompanying artery that must be separately dissected and ligated before the nerve is divided.

Having divided all the muscles around the femur, ligate any remaining vessels and avoid the use of diathermy. Check the exact point of division of the femur and scrape the periosteum from the bone in this region. The thigh muscles must be retracted proximally to give you enough room to use the saw. This can be done with the aid of a couple of abdominal packs or a specially designed retractor.

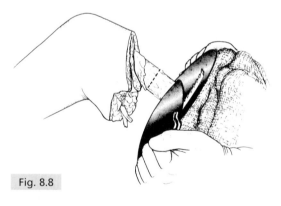

Fig. 8.8

After dividing the femur and removing the lower leg, place clean towels under the stump and rest the stump on an upturned bowl.

Use a rasp to smooth off the edge of the femur and then bring the anterior and posterior muscles together over the bone using an interrupted size 1 absorbable suture. Place a suction drain under the muscle layer. Place a second layer of absorbable sutures more superficially in the muscle and subcutaneous tissues as this will help to approximate the skin flaps. Suture the skin edges with a series of interrupted 2/0 non-absorbable sutures, trying to avoid picking up the edges with toothed forceps. Cover the stump with gauze and cotton-wool dressing and bandage it tightly with crepe bandage.

Below-knee amputation

The optimum site for division is 14 cm from the tibial plateau, the fibula being divided 2 cm proximal to this. Mark out the incision, with the anterior flap ending just distal to the line of bone section on the tibia and the posterior flap extending down to the Achilles tendon.

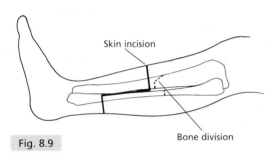

Fig. 8.9

Incise along the marked lines. Posteriorly divide the Achilles tendon and deepen the incision to divide across the remainder of the muscles and tendons down to the bone. Divide the muscles deep to the anterior division transversely.

Cut the fibula obliquely using a Gigli saw and then divide the tibia 2 cm distal to this. Clear the muscle off the bone with a periosteal elevator. Cut an anterior bevel first by sawing diagonally and then cut perpendicularly across the tibia.

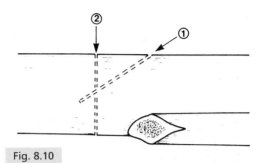

Fig. 8.10

Bevelling the tibia

Angle the lower end of the tibia upwards and separate the muscle mass from its posterior aspect. Double-ligate all vessels and divide any nerves under tension. Remove the distal leg.

Wrap the posterior flap upwards around the bony stump and suture it to the shorter anterior flap. The bulk of the posterior flap may need to be reduced by excision of muscle tissue to achieve this.

Place absorbable sutures between the muscle posteriorly and the subcutaneous tissues anteriorly and leave a suction drain under the muscle. Unite the skin edges with interrupted non-absorbable 2/0 sutures. Trimming the corners of the posterior flap is necessary in order to achieve a good fit. Apply a cotton-wool dressing to the stump and bandage it tightly with crepe.

Key points

1. Amputations may be performed under regional or general anaesthetic.
2. Check and double-check that you are operating on the correct side.
3. Try and isolate areas of gangrene such as the foot with a rubber glove.
4. Make generous flaps since they can always be trimmed back later.
5. If the tissues of an ischaemic limb do not bleed adequately move more proximally with the amputation.
6. Do not suture the drains as this allows them to be removed without undoing the dressings.
7. The dressing can be left undisturbed for 2 weeks. Inspect the wound if the patient complains of excessive pain, has a temperature, or the stump begins to smell.
8. Prescribe prophylactic penicillin if the patient has gangrene.
9. Ensure early mobilisation so that flexion contractures do not develop.

9

HEAD AND NECK

Indications

1. Thyrotoxicosis.
2. Pressure symptoms – dyspnoea, dysphagia.
3. Cosmesis – large multinodular goitre.
4. Malignancy.

Setting up

1. General anaesthesia.
2. Supine with neck extended.
3. Sandbags under shoulders and head ring for support.

Procedure

Mark the skin incision 2 cm above the sternal notch using a heavy suture. Try to place it within an existing skin crease. It is useful to mark parallel lines in the skin using a pen so as to aid alignment at the end of the operation.

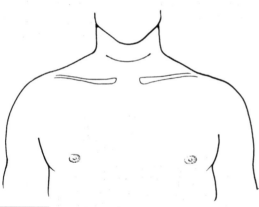

Fig. 9.1

Extend the incision as far laterally as the medial border of sternomastoid and deepen it through platysma.

Place three pairs of tissue forceps on the subcutaneous tissues of the upper flap and elevate the forceps so as to demonstrate the plane for dissection. Using a combination of blunt and sharp dissection separate the flap from the underlying strap muscles.

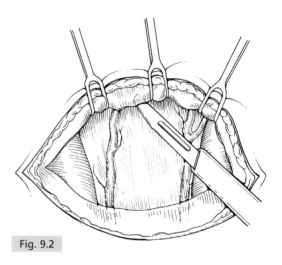

Fig. 9.2

Continue this process superiorly to the upper border of the thyroid cartilage and then repeat inferiorly to the sternal notch.

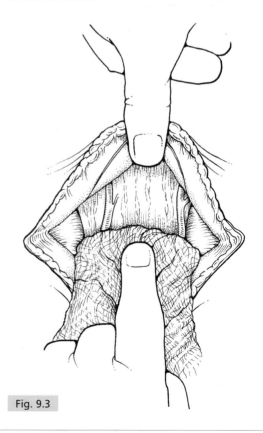

Fig. 9.3

Apply two small wound towels and then a Joll's retractor with its clips at the midpoint of the incision.

Incise and then divide the pretracheal fascia in the midline along the length of the incision. Mobilise medial border of sternomastoid.

Begin dissecting the plane between the strap muscles and the thyroid. Identify, ligate and divide the middle thyroid vein.

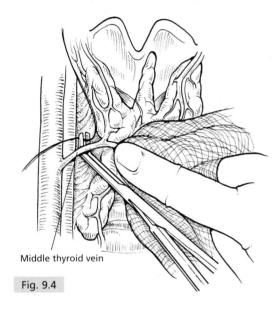

Middle thyroid vein

Fig. 9.4

Proceed cranially, dissecting slowly and carefully to avoid the recurrent laryngeal nerve. Identify the superior thyroid pedicle and pass a Kocher's grooved director underneath it. Feed a heavy tie into the

groove using an aneurysm needle and ligate the pedicle. Repeat the process and then divide the pedicle with a knife.

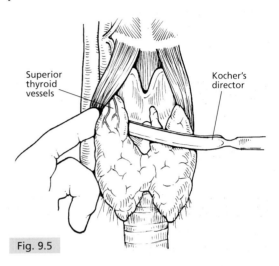

Superior thyroid vessels

Kocher's director

Fig. 9.5

Using a gauze swab to retract the thyroid medially and identify the recurrent laryngeal nerve. Dissect down the lateral aspect of the lobe until the inferior thyroid vessels are found. Ligate and divide the vessels if a thyroid lobectomy is being performed. In the case of a subtotal thyroidectomy they may be preserved.

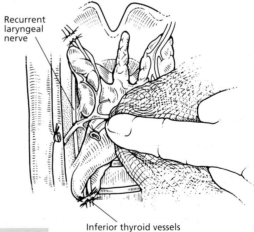

Recurrent laryngeal nerve

Inferior thyroid vessels

Fig. 9.6

In the case of thyroid lobectomy, apply a heavy forceps to the thyroid in the midline, divide the thyroid and oversew the remaining lobe with an absorbable suture, thus removing the isthmus with the specimen.

Secure haemostasis and then insert a small suction drain into the thyroid bed. Bring the drain out between the strap muscles. If the strap muscles were divided, repair them with interrupted absorbable sutures. The platysma may be closed with a continuous absorbable suture.

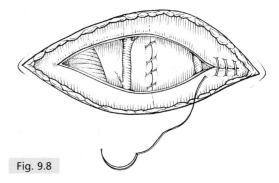

Fig. 9.8

Close the skin with metal clips.

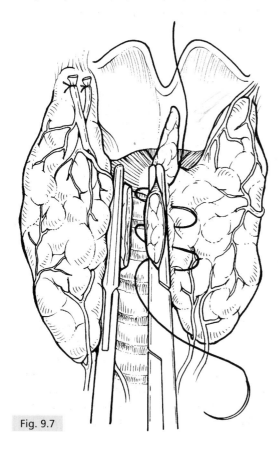

Fig. 9.7

Dissect the thyroid free from the surface of the trachea. Control any bleeding points with fine clips and ligate them individually.

For a subtotal thyroidectomy perform a similar mobilisation to the other lobe. Divide the isthmus and work laterally, freeing the thyroid from the trachea. Apply a series of forceps to the lateral portions of the gland with the aim of leaving approximately 5 cm³. Excise the thyroid with a scalpel and oversew the remnants with a continuous absorbable suture, securing them to the trachea.

Key points

1. A preoperative cord check must be performed.
2. If the goitre is large and access difficult the strap muscles may be ligated and divided.
3. Make sure you identify the correct plane for dissection. Failure to do so will result in an obscured operating field.
4. When ligating the superior pedicle keep towards the thyroid so as not to damage the external laryngeal nerve.
5. Always identify and avoid the recurrent laryngeal nerve as it runs along the lateral border of the gland.
6. Try not to damage the parathyroids or their blood supply from the inferior thyroid artery.
7. Always have a pair of clip removers at hand on the ward in case the patient develops a haematoma, as this may cause respiratory obstruction.

Indications

1. Cosmesis.
2. Recurrent infection – in the presence of infection treat with antibiotics and excise after 4–6 weeks.

Setting up

1. General anaesthetic.
2. Prone position with neck extended.
3. Sandbags under shoulders and head ring for support.

Procedure

Make a transverse incision over the cyst and deepen the incision through the subcutaneous tissues and platysma.

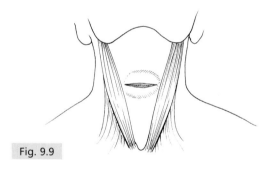

Fig. 9.9

Divide and ligate the anterior jugular veins as they pass over the midline. Identify the cyst and sharply dissect away from the surrounding tissue, taking care not to puncture the cyst.

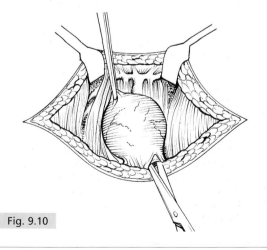

Fig. 9.10

Place a pair of tissue forceps on the cyst and apply traction caudally. Dissect the tract up to the hyoid bone and free the muscle attachments and thyrohyoid membrane. Isolate the central portion of the hyoid and excise it in continuity with the tract and cyst using heavy scissors or bone cutters (Sistrunk's procedure).

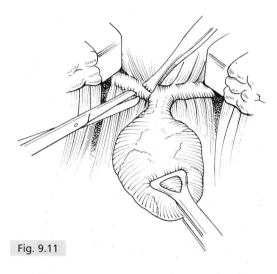

Fig. 9.11

Examine for any tract passing from the superior border of the hyoid towards the tongue and excise if present, closing the duct proximally with an absorbable suture. Obtain haemostasis with bipolar diathermy and insert a small suction drain. Close the subcutaneous tissue with an absorbable suture and the skin with a subcuticular absorbable suture.

Key points

1. Take care not to puncture the thyrohyoid membrane when dividing the hyoid.
2. Ensure that the hyoid bone is excised, as failure to do so predisposes to recurrence.

10

UROLOGICAL

CIRCUMCISION

Indications

1. Infants   Recurrent balanitis.
               Phimosis
               Religious or cultural reasons.
2. Adults   Recurrent balanitis.
               Paraphimosis.
               Underlying tumour on the glans penis.

Setting up

1. General anaesthetic with dorsal block.
2. Supine position.

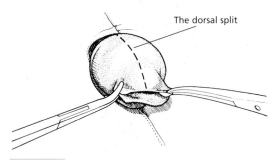

The dorsal split

Fig. 10.1

Procedure

Grasp the prepuce on each side with mosquito clips and make a dorsal slit with a scissors.

This dorsal slit procedure can be used to facilitate urethral catheterisation in the presence of a phimosis in the elderly male.

Carefully separate any attachments to the glans penis and clean any retained secretions. Extend the dorsal slit down towards the corona. Make a careful ventral slit up to the frenulum.

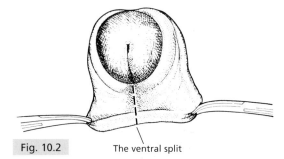

Fig. 10.2   The ventral split

Secure the frenular artery with an absorbable suture, leaving one end long.

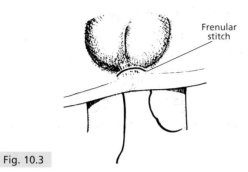

Frenular stitch

Fig. 10.3

The prepuce, which is now in two halves, can be excised with scissors, maintaining some tension on the frenular stitch.

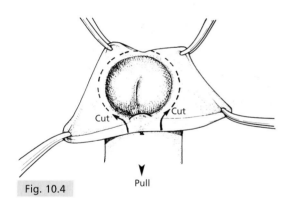

Cut Cut

Fig. 10.4

Pull

Ligate any individual bleeding vessels with fine absorbable sutures and then suture the skin edges to the mucosa with interrupted absorbable sutures commencing at 3, 6, 9 and 12 o'clock positions and then infilling the gaps between these sutures.

The final 6 o'clock suture can be used to hold the penis whilst a dressing is applied. Smear the wound with lignocaine gel. A conventional 'sporran' dressing is the easiest to manage.

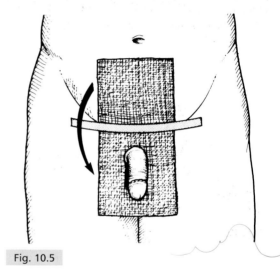

Fig. 10.5

Key points

1. Do not leave too much skin – about 0.5 cm around the glans penis is satisfactory.
2. Be careful to avoid the meatus when doing the initial dorsal slit.
3. Always warn parents that during healing the appearance can appear slightly alarming, but that once the crusting has disappeared healing will be satisfactory.
4. Try and avoid the use of diathermy. If necessary use bipolar diathermy.
5. This procedure is ideal for day-case surgery.

Indications

Male sterilization – conventionally between the ages of 28 and 45, with a stable marriage and a family of two or more children.

Setting up

1. Local anaesthetic.
2. Supine position.

Procedure

The secret of this operation is to locate and fix the vas with one hand until it can be grasped with an instrument through the incision with the other hand. Standing on the patient's right, feel for either vas in the upper scrotum with the thumb of your non-dominant hand behind it, and the index and middle fingers over the anterior surface of it.

Infiltrate the skin with 1% lignocaine and introduce further local anaesthetic into the coverings of the vas itself.

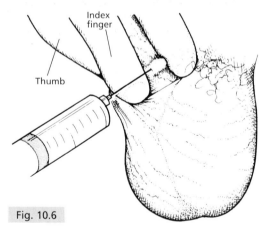

Fig. 10.6

Infiltrate both the skin and the vas

Make a small incision along the vas and with gentle dissection identify the vas in the incision. Using a cross-action towel clip grasp the vas and dissect it from its coverings with a scalpel along its line. It is important to get down onto the plane of the vas itself in order to be able to free-up enough length.

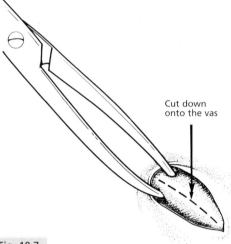

Cut down onto the vas

Fig. 10.7

Excise a segment of vas about a centimetre long and send it for histological confirmation.

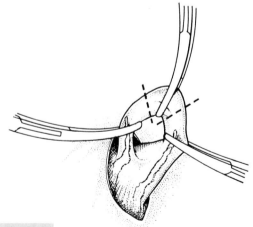

Fig. 10.8

Tie the base of the vas.

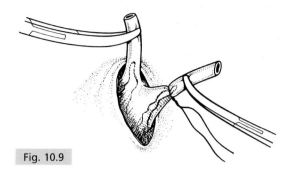

Fig. 10.9

Then double over each of the cut ends and ligate a second time.

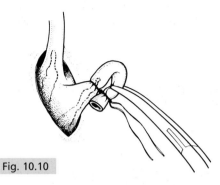

Fig. 10.10

Close the incision with interrupted absorbable sutures before repeating the procedure on the contralateral vas.

Key points

1. It is important to counsel both partners prior to the operation, mentioning the irreversibility of the procedure and the necessity for two consecutive azoospermic counts after the operation. Also mention the reasons for failure, which can be technical at the initial operation or due to re-cannalisation of the vas subsequently.

Indications

Symptomatic swelling in adults.

Setting up

1. General anaesthetic.
2. Supine position.

Procedure

Stretch the scrotum over the anterior aspect of the hydrocele with the non-dominant hand and incise between any visible vessels using either a knife or cutting diathermy.

Make a small incision in the tunica vaginalis and evacuate the fluid. Enlarge the hole with the scissors until it is big enough to allow the testis to be removed from the hemi-scrotum. Check that the testis is normal.

Two main techniques are used for hydrocele repair:

Jaboulay

Using absorbable sutures stitch the edges of the tunica behind the cord and subsequently return the testis to the scrotum.

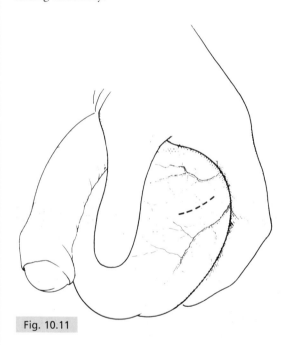

Fig. 10.11

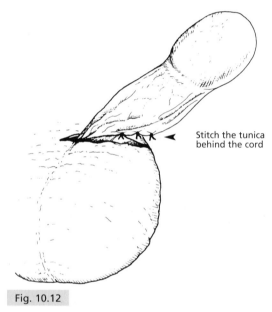

Stitch the tunica behind the cord

Fig. 10.12

Lord's procedure

Using a series of interrupted catgut sutures bunch-up the remaining sac around the testis before tying the sutures and returning the testis to the scrotum. Remember that in order to return the testis to the scrotum you will need to create a space by blunt dissection with the fingers.

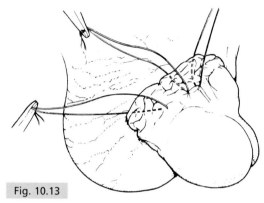

Fig. 10.13

Place all the sutures before tying them

Haemostasis is extremely important. Spend a little time achieving this before suturing the wound.

Close the skin with interrupted absorbable sutures.

Key points

1. Remember in men under the age of 35–40 to think of testicular tumour – preoperative ultrasound can be helpful.
2. In the elderly and chronically sick, repeated needle aspiration may be more appropriate.
3. Blood in hydrocele is found on trauma, torsion and some testicular tumours, so be aware of this when aspirating hydroceles.
4. The technique in a child is the same as that for an infantile inguinal herniotomy (p. 22). As a rule it is unnecessary to operate on infantile hydroceles unless they persist beyond 18 months to 2 years of age.

Indications

1. Male infertility.
2. Aching and discomfort in the scrotum.

Several techniques are available for the treatment of varicocele:

- Radiological embolisation.
- Laparoscopic division of the varicocele from within the peritoneal cavity.
- Surgical approach to the varicocele at the level of the internal ring.

Only the latter approach will be described here.

Setting up

1. General anaesthetic.
2. Supine position.

Procedure

The varicocele is usually left-sided. Make an incision over the internal ring, parallel to the inguinal ligament.

Divide the external oblique aponeurosis, visualise the cord and split the spermatic fascia longitudinally to allow the large testicular veins to become visible.

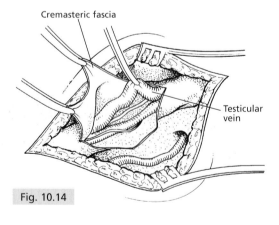

Cremasteric fascia

Testicular vein

Fig. 10.14

Separate the veins from the vas and the testicular artery and, after division, ligate with an absorbable suture.

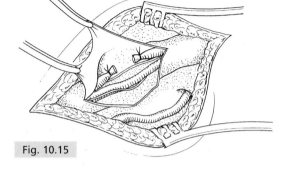

Fig. 10.15

Repair the external oblique aponeurosis with an absorbable suture and close the skin incision with a subcuticular non-absorbable suture.

Key points

1. An acute onset of left varicocele can occur as a presentation of renal cell tumour on the left side, but varicoceles are generally fairly common.
2. Varicoceles are associated with oligospermia.

Indications

Larger and uncomfortable cysts.

Setting up

1. General anaesthetic.
2. Supine position.

Procedure

Using your non-dominant hand stretch the scrotal skin over the anterior aspect of the hydrocele. Identify any small vessels and incise between them (Fig. 10.11).

Evacuate the fluid by making a small incision in the tunica vaginalis and enlarge this until it is adequate for exteriorisation of the testis.

Using artery clips deliver the testis and epididymis through the scrotal incision. Excise the cysts, which are often multiple, and return the testis to the scrotum.

Transfix the redundant cyst wall with an absorbable suture. Be careful to maintain haemostasis and close the incision with an interrupted absorbable suture.

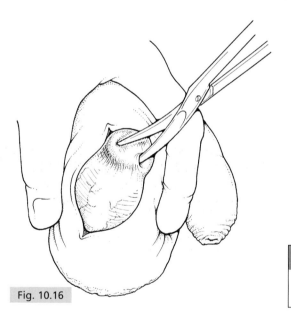

Fig. 10.16

Key point

1. Clear fluid implies an epididymal cyst whereas white fluid implies a spermatocele.

Indications

An undescended testis in a child.

Setting up

1. General anaesthetic.
2. Supine position.

Procedure

Make a 3 cm incision in the inguinal skin crease.

The testis is usually found in the region of the external ring; a little proximal pressure above the ring can cause the testis to appear if it is not immediately obvious.

Incise the external oblique aponeurosis, gently pick up the testis and divide the gubernaculum testis.

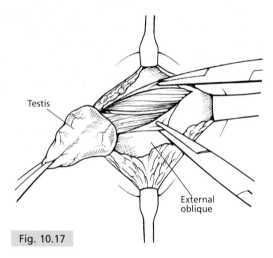

Testis

External
oblique

Fig. 10.17

Mobilise the cord sufficiently to allow the testis to reach the scrotum. Achieve this by dividing the bands that are attached to the cord laterally and medially, taking care to preserve the vas and the testicular vessels.

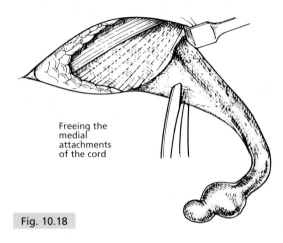

Freeing the
medial
attachments
of the cord

Fig. 10.18

Identify the hernial sac which is often present. Carefully dissect this off the cord, ligate and divide it at the internal ring.

Prepare the scrotum by passing a finger down into it and making a transverse incision in the scrotal skin over the tip of the finger.

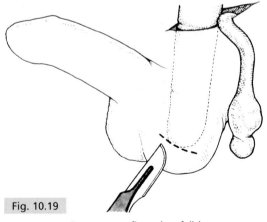

Fig. 10.19

Cut onto your finger (carefully)

Leave the layer of fascia covering the finger and, by spreading the blades of a pair of scissors, prepare a subdartos pouch between this fascia and the overlying skin. Push the points of the forceps onto your finger so that they pierce the fascial layer and, as your finger is withdrawn, pass the forceps up towards the inguinal wound to grasp the testis.

Carefully pull the testis down into the scrotum, easing it through the defect in the fascia.

Anchor the testis to the dartos muscle with an interrupted absorbable suture and close the scrotal skin with a similar suture. Close the groin wound with a continuous absorbable suture to the external oblique and a subcuticular absorbable suture to the skin.

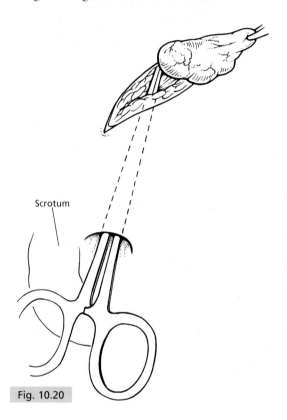

Scrotum

Fig. 10.20

Key points

1. Remember that some 30% of premature infants have maldescent on both sides, and 3% of full-term infants have maldescent at birth.
2. An empty scrotal sac may imply that the testis is absent, retractile, ectopic or maldescended.
3. If you can't get the testicle to reach the scrotum despite your best efforts, call for help. If help is not available, place the testis as low down as you can and plan for a subsequent procedure when the child is older.
4. If the testis is not present make sure that you look within the inguinal canal; but a subsequent laparoscopy may become necessary.
5. Most orchidopexies should be done between the ages of 2 and 3.

Indications

Suspected torsion.

Setting up

1. General anaesthetic.
2. Supine position.

Procedure

Approach the testis through a scrotal incision.

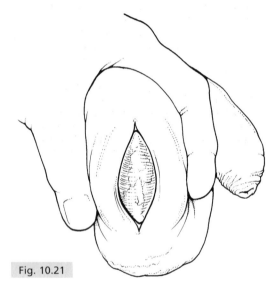

Fig. 10.21

Open the tunica vaginalis, inspect and untwist the torsion.

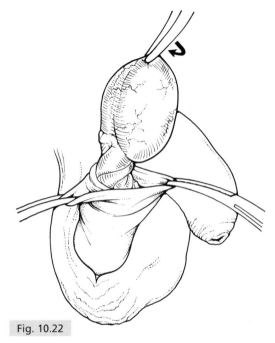

Fig. 10.22

Wrap the testicle in moist warm swabs and, if the testis appears viable, return it to the scrotum. It is always better to err on the side of caution rather than to excise the testis unnecessarily. If, however, the testicle is necrotic, apply a crushing clamp and transfix and ligate the cord and then excise the testis.

Fix the testis to the tunica vaginalis with three anchoring sutures, one at each pole and one at the centre.

If a torsion is found, fix the contralateral testis prophylactically in a similar manner.

Close the incision with interrupted absorbable sutures.

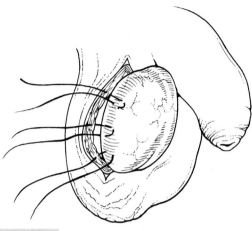

Fig. 10.23

Key points

1. When the diagnosis of testicular torsion is made or even suspected, immediate exploration is indicated within 8 hours. After 8 hours the infarcted testis is unlikely to recovery.
2. Remember that neonates can have testicular torsion which often presents at birth with a red, non-tender scrotal mass.
3. In a suspected torsion, remember that undescended testes tort more than normal testes and that a painful undescended testis can imply a torsion.
4. It is difficult to distinguish clinically between testicular torsion and torsion of the appendages of the testis. If torsion of an appendage is found, excise the lesion. In this case contralateral exploration is not indicated.

INDEX